a safe place for women

Kelly White has led programs that raise funds and provide services for ending violence against women and children. She has been the CEO at the Chicago Foundation for Women, SafePlace in Austin, and the Austin Children's Shelter. Kelly is a formerly battered woman who strives to bring a human face to a problem that is still shrouded in shame and secrecy. She has escaped to a shelter, dealt with the criminal-justice system, and juggled the many competing priorities of a single mom, and she has always brought these experiences to her work.

"The book *A Safe Place for Women* is a primer on domestic violence and the organizations that exist to help victims. This book should be required reading for all board members of domestic-violence shelters."
— Julia Spann, Executive Director of SafePlace

"Kelly White's unique perspective as a survivor, activist, and service provider gives her readers a complex portrait of dreams gone awry and resilience in the face of hardship. We need a book like hers to give hope to the millions of women who suffer abuse and inspiration to those wanting to create a safer world."
— Sunny Fischer, Co-founder of the Chicago Foundation
for Women and antiviolence activist

"Kelly White provides a compelling and heroic personal and professional account of survivorship and triumph. Her insights into the impact of trauma and the resolve that exist deeply within humans are brilliant. She describes a process where healing is possible. Her story is beautifully documented and is a must read for all of us who are committed to and care about our families and members of our communities."
— Noël Bridget Busch-Armendariz, PhD, LMSW, MPA
Associate Professor and Director, School of Social Work,
Institute on Domestic Violence & Sexual Assault

Ordering
Trade bookstores in the U.S. and Canada please contact:

Publishers Group West
1700 Fourth Street, Berkeley CA 94710
Phone: (800) 788-3123   Fax: (800) 351-5073

Hunter House books are available at bulk discounts for textbook course adoptions;
to qualifying community, health-care, and government organizations;
and for special promotions and fund-raising. For details please contact:

Special Sales Department
Hunter House Inc., PO Box 2914, Alameda CA 94501-0914
Phone: (510) 865-5282   Fax: (510) 865-4295
E-mail: ordering@hunterhouse.com

Individuals can order our books from most bookstores,
by calling **(800) 266-5592**, or from our website at
www.hunterhouse.com

a safe place for women

Surviving Domestic Abuse and Creating a Successful Future

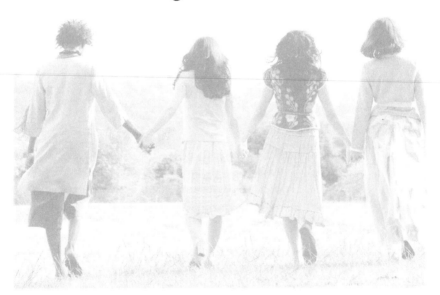

kelly white

Hunter House
PUBLISHERS

Hunter House Inc., Publishers
PO Box 2914
Alameda CA 94501-0914

Library of Congress Cataloging-in-Publication Data
White, Kelly.
A safe place for women : surviving domestic abuse
and creating a successful future / Kelly White.
p.   cm.
Includes index.
ISBN 978-0-89793-527-2
1. Abused women.   2. Family violence.   3. Family violence—Prevention.
4. Victims of family violence.   I. Title.
HV6626.W484 2010
362.82'92–dc22   2010007020

Project Credits

Cover Design   BRIAN DITTMAR DESIGN, INC.
Book Production   JOHN MCKERCHER
Developmental Editors   ALLAN CREIGHTON and JUDE BERMAN
Copy Editor   KELLEY BLEWSTER
Proofreader   JOHN DAVID MARION
Indexer   CANDACE HYATT
Managing Editor   ALEXANDRA MUMMERY
Senior Marketing Associate   REINA SANTANA
Publicity Coordinator   SEAN HARVEY
Rights Coordinator   CANDACE GROSKREUTZ
Customer Service Manager   CHRISTINA SVERDRUP
Order Fulfillment   WASHUL LAKDHON
Administrator   THERESA NELSON
Computer Support   PETER EICHELBERGER
Publisher   KIRAN S. RANA

Printed and bound by Bang Printing, Brainerd, Minnesota
Manufactured in the United States of America

9 8 7 6 5 4 3 2 1   First Edition   11 12 13 14 15

Contents

Foreword

By Luci Baines Johnson

Parts of Kelly White's life story are all too familiar. Tragically, domestic violence is an equal-opportunity scourge on the American landscape. It affects rich and poor, young and old, black, brown, and white, male and female, straight and gay, famous and your next-door neighbor.

Kelly's story is about a young mother's anguishing experience with this national epidemic, her escape into a safe, productive life, and, ultimately, her respectful and loving marriage to a man who considers her a full partner, lover, and friend.

What makes Kelly's story special is how she's used her experience to help countless others escape the pain she once knew. Like many victims of domestic violence Kelly fled the marriage, taking her two young sons across the country into a new life. But Kelly's new life also included helping others escape from domestic violence. Eventually, she led the transformation of the Center for Battered Women, in Austin, Texas, by merging it with the Austin Rape Crisis Center to create SafePlace, which became a national model for working to end rape, sexual abuse, and domestic violence.

It was at the Center for Battered Women that I first met Kelly.

I was there because I, too, needed a way to turn my heartache into something good.

My life has been deeply blessed. As President Lyndon Baines Johnson's daughter, I've had the opportunity to be an eyewitness to history and meet many of the movers and shakers of my time. But, sadly, I've also seen the anguish of domestic violence. My dearest childhood friend, a bridesmaid at my White House wedding, was murdered by her husband. Domestic violence affects even our nation's first families.

I met Kelly in another time of economic stress—the early nineties. Kelly was serving as director of the Center for Battered Women in Austin, my hometown. She knew that the need for domestic-violence and rape-crisis services increases during the financial stress of recession. She recognized the economic benefits that could be realized for each organization by merging them.

Kelly was instrumental in awakening the conscience of residents of Central Texas to the needs of survivors of domestic violence and rape. Whenever Austin had a civic meeting, Kelly was there. She located every governmental, corporate, and individual dollar that was available to address the problems of violence against women and children. She enlisted others in support of her innovative ideas, making Austin's program one of the nation's leaders in the intervention and prevention of domestic violence, sexual abuse, and rape.

I had the honor of serving with hundreds of others in Kelly's mighty army.

She motivated me, and many others, to think bigger. She helped us believe that we could and should work to merge rape and domestic-violence services, build residential apartments on the campus of a domestic-violence center, provide an elementary school on campus — and the list goes on.

Who will benefit from reading *A Safe Place for Women*? Anyone who believes that with hard work and commitment to community the most difficult problems can be solved. Anyone whose family has been touched by domestic violence. Anyone who works to end the plague of violence against women, and anyone who wants to make a difference. This is a story of America at its best.

— Luci Baines Johnson

Luci Baines Johnson, daughter of US President Lyndon Johnson and his wife, Ladybird, is Chairman of the Board of the LBJ Holding Company and serves on the Board of Trustees of the SafePlace Foundation. Luci's passion for ending domestic violence was generated by the murder of her grade-school friend, a bridesmaid at her White House wedding, who was shot and killed by her husband.

Acknowledgments

A special thank you to my sister Jacqueline White Kochak, who gave of her expertise, her talent, and her time to help me organize and put all of my disparate thoughts onto paper. A special thank you also to my dear friend and colleague Julia Spann, who has read, reread, edited, written, reminded, encouraged, and generally held my hand.

It is impossible not to recognize the women and men of SafePlace in Austin, Texas. I have been blessed to work with the most extraordinary group of people who daily make a difference in the lives of countless others. I have received much credit over the years simply because I have been the one out front telling the stories while my colleagues were behind the scenes doing the real work of changing and saving lives. This book is dedicated to the employees, volunteers, board members, donors, and clients who have nurtured and created a safe place for so many. I want to particularly acknowledge Diane McDaniel Rhodes, Melinda Cantu, Wendie Abramson, Barri Rosenbluth, Sue Snyder, Linda Herbert, LeeAnn Cameron, Gail Rice, Ellen Fisher, Angela Atwood, Erin Clark, and Karen Wilson.

Important Note

The material in this book is intended to provide a review of information regarding resources for survivors of domestic abuse. Every effort has been made to provide accurate and dependable information. The contents of this book have been compiled through professional research and in consultation with medical and mental-health professionals. However, professionals have differing opinions, and advances in research are made very quickly, so some of the information may become outdated.

Therefore, the publisher, author, and editors, as well as the professionals quoted in the book, cannot be held responsible for any error, omission, or dated material. The authors and publisher assume no responsibility for any outcome of applying the information in this book in a program of self-care or under the care of a licensed practitioner. If you have questions concerning the application of the information described in this book, consult a qualified mental-health or legal professional.

introduction

TWENTY YEARS AFTER I FIRST SOUGHT REFUGE IN A BATTERED women's shelter, I stood under a tent in Austin, Texas, surrounded by hundreds of friends and supporters as the chair of the Austin Safe-Place board of directors announced, to my absolute incredulity, that the 105-bed shelter I had led the effort to build was being named the Kelly White Family Shelter in my honor.

I have chosen to tell my story, intertwined with the story of Safe-Place, because it is the story I know best. It is a story that could be told in many different communities, using many different names, across the country and around the world. My destiny has been to give a face and a voice to battered women. I first spoke out publicly as a formerly battered woman in the early 1980s when a reporter at a press conference asked, "Why is it that all we ever hear from is you women who run these shelters who are telling us it's such a big problem? Why don't we ever hear from the battered women?"

In that moment I realized I needed to step forward as a formerly battered woman who ran a shelter and give a face to the issue — the face of a white, educated, middle-class mom who didn't fit the existing stereotype of a poor minority or a so-called man-hating "feminazi." Instead, I was a woman who wore panty hose and makeup, shaved her legs, and looked forward to someday having a loving and fulfilling relationship with a good man. I was the face that had been hidden behind closed doors for too long.

I have been stepping forward ever since. I now live a great life by almost anyone's standards. I have three well-adjusted children, all grown or nearly so, and I am happily married to Bill McLellan, a smart, funny, successful, and, most importantly, respectful man who adores me. He said he hoped to get a mention in the last chapter, but I realized he needed a mention right up front, since it is largely because of him that I had the time, the freedom, and the financial wherewithal to take on the rather daunting task of writing a book.

I have a life that is better than anything I ever dreamed of. However, it is only over the last two decades that I have learned how to dream and to expect the best for myself. I have learned that I deserve love, support, and success.

This book is much more than a personal memoir; it details violence against women and children from my unique perspective, as a formerly battered woman who has spent more than twenty years helping other women and children to survive.

My stepping forward includes writing this book and telling the inspirational stories of survivors. Through the stories, I hope to help others understand why and how battering occurs and how each of us can recognize it and work for change. This book is intended for survivors of battering, for their friends and loved ones — for anyone who is trying to understand the realities of domestic violence and the issues surrounding it. The final three chapters are more specifically written for practitioners, the thousands of individuals who work in the field. I am a survivor and I have worked in the field for over two decades, but I am quick to acknowledge that I am not, nor have I ever been, an expert in providing direct support and services for battered women. My expertise lies in figuring out how to make the programs work, including finding the all-too-necessary money to keep the doors open, and in telling survivors' stories. My most cherished hope is that others, by reading this book, will realize the continuing need for policy change, allied services, and — yes — additional funding.

Throughout the book I use several terms interchangeably: domestic violence, intimate-partner violence, battering, and family violence. These terms are generally used to describe a pattern of behavior that includes verbal, emotional, economic, physical, and/or sexual abuse. Most importantly, they portray a pattern of behavior in any relationship that is used to gain or maintain power and control over an intimate partner. Rarely, however, does battering or domestic violence follow an orderly progression from one type of abuse to another.

I have known women who were killed by their husbands when they tried to leave emotionally and verbally abusive marriages. Police records note, "There was no history of domestic violence," because there were no prior physical assaults. But these women knew the potential outcome all too well. They had been repeatedly told, "If you try to leave me, I will kill you." Although they may have been physically assaulted only once — the assault that led to their death — these women were battered in every sense of the word. I have also known women who have never been physically assaulted, and may never be, but have endured such persistent and destructive assaults on their self-esteem that they will forever live under the thumb of their abusive partner.

I have changed the names and identifying characteristics of many people in the book to protect their privacy. When only a first name is listed, I am likely using a pseudonym. If both a first and last name are stated, I want the person to be recognized and applauded for the work they have done and the obstacles they have overcome. I have changed my ex-husband's name out of respect for our sons and because I know that he has worked hard to try to build a new life for himself.

"We hoped it would be different this time," his family said to me after our divorce. I knew he had been married before, but I had never been told of the problems with violence that led his first wife to leave the marriage and the state. I also know that he had to deal with problems associated with his violent behavior in a relationship after our marriage. However, he is not an "evil" man; he is a man who battles his own furious demons.

I once loved him enough to marry him, and there were times when grief over the loss of our marriage and the dream of what could have/should have been was powerful enough to bring me to my knees, wails of despair originating deep in my gut. How does one explain the profound mourning over the loss of a fairy tale, the loss of the idealized marriage and family that I'd built in my mind and that I'd fervently believed, if I just tried hard enough, I could make work.

One of the most difficult things for people to understand is the complex love–hate relationship a battered woman often has with her abusive partner. The day I stood in court for my final divorce decree, I remember saying to the judge that, more than anything, I just wanted my ex-husband to be "okay." I wanted him to be the good and supportive husband and the caring and involved father the sitcoms of the sixties and seventies seemed to promise. I just wanted the battering to stop.

I had married a handsome man. I was drawn to his movie-star good looks; when we walked down the street, all heads would turn to watch him pass. He was tall and lean with thick dark hair and piercing blue-gray eyes. I was also drawn to his intelligence; he was smart and seemed capable of doing anything he set his mind to. He was sensitive, a gifted painter and artist. Here, I thought, was a man who had enormous potential, and it seemed to me at the time that he just needed me to help him be whole.

I am a "fixer" and a "healer." I majored in occupational therapy in college because I wanted to help people heal. I have spent my entire life "fixing" houses, organizations, gardens, and anything else I can get my hands on. So it was very difficult for me to give up the belief that if I just tried harder I could fix or heal my marriage. When I finally learned to let go of the belief that I could change my husband, I also learned to let others help me heal. Through this lesson I have met the most extraordinary people.

It is impossible for me to mention the thousands of people I have worked with over the years who've made a difference in my life and the lives of the women and children from SafePlace and similar programs. I have tried to recall circumstances and conversations as accurately as possible and to convey their essence honestly, while of necessity reconstructing some events and discussions.

Time has a wondrous curative effect. Many of the memories of some of my most frightening moments are blurred around the edges. I think this may be a mechanism our minds use to help us heal and function. But if the exact timing or circumstances of a memory are slightly off, the larger picture is always correct.

Why am I writing a book that is intensely personal in so many ways? First of all, in over twenty-five years of working with and for battered women and their children, I have met a whole world full of heroes whose stories should be told. I have met women, children, and men who have overcome enormous hardship, sometimes even tragedy, and turned their experiences toward helping others.

Second, I have seen abysmal failures in the systems charged with protecting us. Our families, the medical community, criminal-justice programs, educational institutions, churches, mental-health facilities, and many more, do not always function as they could. Some of these failures have tragic consequences that can reverberate across generations. I would like to see this change.

Finally, I am writing this book because there is so much work to be done. Our shelters are still full, mothers still return with their children to abusive husbands just so their children will have homes, and women still don't have the status — around the world and right here in our country — to overcome abuse and thrive.

We still live in a world plagued by female sexual slavery in Thailand, the mass raping of women in countries engaged in war, female genital mutilation in Africa, and widow burnings, dowry deaths, and selective forced abortions in India and China. These represent only a few of the many human rights violations that are inflicted upon women simply because of their gender. It continues to be dangerous just to be a girl.

The predominant culture in the United States continues to be one of patriarchy, and acceptance of violence is pervasive. In some communities its growth is exponential. The popular media often promulgate misogyny and violence against women, and females are portrayed in objectified and sexualized ways.

Clearly, our work isn't nearly done. We have, however, accomplished more than anyone thought possible. When my ex-husband stalked me in the early eighties, I was told there was nothing law enforcement could do until he actually hurt me. Not a very comforting situation. Now, women in similar situations can almost always turn to law enforcement officers because stalking laws are, for the most part, universal in the United States. In most municipalities and states, the laws have been changed so that a woman no longer has to fight to have charges pressed against her batterer. The responding law enforcement officer can charge him with assault and jail him. Unfortunately, individual officers are not always responsive, and our overcrowded court system is often ineffective at best, and injurious at worst.

Of course, we now also have a network of battered women's and rape crisis programs across the nation, every one of which continues to be underfunded and overburdened with clients. But twenty years ago you were lucky if your community had a shelter at all.

I am writing this book because it is a story that should be told, the story of a movement created from the ground up, the story of the lives that have been saved because of the passion, sweat, and sacrifice of those who cared enough to take on the system and to create something from nothing.

The story of SafePlace and my story as a survivor of domestic violence both began in the mid-1970s, a time when battered-women's and rape-crisis programs were just being started across the nation. No one had even heard the term "violence against women." When I hear politicians and others speak longingly of the good old days — the 1950s and 1960s, the time of the nuclear family, with moms at home cooking, cleaning, and caring for the kids, and dads at work supporting the family — I am amazed at how much was hidden behind those "happy" façades. Domestic violence, incest, and rape were rarely acknowledged, and the victim was often blamed for being "flirtatious," "bitchy," or "provocative." In other words, they were somehow responsible for their own black eyes, broken bones, and wounded psyches. When the first women's centers were started, the founders were shunned as being "man-haters" while simultaneously being astonished at the number of women who came forward seeking safety and shelter from their so-called idyllic homes. Thus began a movement.

SafePlace was started in Austin in 1977 as the Center for Battered Women. It was the first battered women's shelter in Texas and one of the first twenty in the nation. Like most programs of its type, it was started by a committed group of feminists. Many of these same women had come together a few years earlier to start the Austin Rape Crisis Center. Twenty years later, the two programs merged to become SafePlace, which eventually grew into an internationally recognized model for providing domestic-violence and sexual-assault services. In addition, many of these same pioneering women also started the Texas Council on Family Violence, from which grew the National Domestic Violence Hotline, a twenty-four-hour, state-of-the-art service that answers almost a quarter of a million calls annually.

I am often asked why Austin would have one of the largest domestic-violence and sexual-assault programs in the nation. Is there more violence against women in Central Texas? Of course not! Austin is a unique community for Texas, a bright blue city in a sea of conservative red. It is nestled among the rolling hills and lakes of Central Texas and is billed the Live Music Capital of the World. An educational Mecca, Austin boasts seven major universities and two seminaries within a thirty-five-mile radius. For many years state government and the University of Texas defined the city. Already the home of Dell Computers and Whole Foods Market, Austin in recent years has seen its economy expand to include high tech and clean energy. It has a diverse, highly educated population with representation from every major world religion.

From the beginning, the people of Austin embraced these programs. SafePlace, and the Center for Battered Women before it, received volunteer and financial support at a level unprecedented for organizations often dismissed elsewhere as "women's programs." Also important to the growth of SafePlace is the fact that it is the only agency of its type in Travis County. The timing of the emergence and growth of battered-women's and rape-crisis programs coincided exactly with the rapid population growth of the Central Texas region. And with the merger of the Austin Rape Crisis Center and the Center for Battered Women, the leaders of the respective agencies, recognizing the needs of clients and the community, ensured an economy of scale in administration and fund-raising. In many other cities, multiple agencies provide the same or similar services, competing for limited dollars and media attention.

No, there isn't more domestic violence in Austin than in other cities. Rather, the Central Texas community stepped forward to address the problem and create innovative solutions. The people of Austin, as well as those who founded and sustained the agency, have made SafePlace special. I believe their story, too, should be told. However, my story and the story of violence against women and children began much earlier. How, I have wondered, do I tell a story that encompasses millions and spans generations? I decided to start where I have always started: with my own.

1

my story: surviving an abusive marriage

My life had been taken from me. I thought I had let it happen and that only I was to blame. My feelings were dead. My self-esteem was dead. And I exposed my slow, tortuous death to my children. I felt I had no place to go. I was trying to arrange everything minute-by-minute, to avoid being punished for what I had come to believe about myself—that I was stupid, that I couldn't manage the simplest of tasks, that I was a bad mother, an incompetent wife, a sexual block of ice. That I was less than dirt and deserved what my husband was dishing out to me.

I came to realize that I wasn't alone, I wasn't crazy, I wasn't worthless. I hadn't done anything "wrong," and the abuse wasn't "my fault." I began to learn that life wasn't something you just let happen to you. I began to learn that you can have some control over your life. You can learn to expect the best, instead of the worst. I have learned that I deserve the best and it's okay to accept it. I have learned that the more I do for my personal development, the better mother I become.

—A formerly battered woman

T HE YEAR WAS 1982 AND THE PLACE WAS LARAMIE, WYOMING, my home for the previous five years. I owned my house, loved my job, and had many good friends. I also had an ex-husband who stalked and harassed me, and who, even after our divorce, managed to control my every move through constant surveillance, bullying, threats, and intimidation. I erroneously believed that by rarely going out with either male or female friends, keeping my family from visiting me, and being at home to answer the phone when he called or drove by at any time of the day or night, I could control the situation. I thought I could maintain the degree of threat at a "manageable" level. But on this particular spring morning my carefully constructed house of cards was toppling around me.

I stood at a pay phone outside a convenience store; my sons, ages three months and two years, were in the backseat of my bright red Toyota Corolla. I had bought the car new just two years before, but now it sported dented fenders, a cracked windshield, and ripped upholstery. The car was one of many objects that all too often bore the brunt of attacks directed at me by Jay, my ex-husband. Those attacks sometimes included potentially deadly kicks and punches; Jay held a black belt in karate. At one point after our divorce he rammed into my car with his pickup truck as my sons and I tried to escape from him by driving across a vacant field. I felt I was at his mercy, my small Corolla no match for his four-wheel-drive pickup on the rutted terrain. Luckily, I was able to drive away when he exited his truck to come after me on foot.

On that day in 1982 I had received a call at work from Jay's counselor, who met with him daily in an effort to manage his out-of-control anger and continuing substance abuse. "Get your children and get to a safe place," he said frantically. "Go now — don't go home first and *do not* go to a friend or family member's home. He knows where to look for you, and he could end up hurting others as well as you. This time you've got to call the battered women's shelter."

At the time I was the executive director of the Developmental Preschool and Daycare, a large nonprofit agency. Our services included a child-care program combined with educational and therapeutic assistance for infants and children with developmental delays. Jay and I had lived apart for at least a year (we had separated while I was pregnant with our second son), and as a single mom I was blessed to be able to bring my children to work with me. I was able to walk down the hall to nurse my baby when he was hungry. I was also lucky to be able to run down the hall and grab my children when I needed to get them to safety.

After receiving that call I raced through the building, mentally calculating how long it would take for Jay to arrive at his apartment, get his gun, and drive to my office. I knew I had mere minutes to snatch my purse and keys, grab my sons, hurry them to the car, buckle them into their car seats, and get all of us out of sight before Jay turned the corner on the far side of the park across the street.

I was terrified, aware that each second ticking away decreased my chance of escaping. And even if I got safely away from the building, Laramie was a small town. Jay could easily find me by driving the streets and looking for my car. Still, minutes later, I stood at a payphone outside the 7-11 where I usually stopped to get my daily Big Gulp. The warm spring morning seemed like a celebration of life after the frigid Wyoming winter, but I was anything but joyous. I was making a call to the SAFE Project, Laramie's battered women's shelter.

I knew the phone number; I had carried a dog-eared card in my wallet for months, perhaps years. I had picked it up at an information table set up outside a store, knowing I might need it one day. The brochure to which the card was attached told about a woman who, like me, thought she could control her husband's rage and abuse until the day he angrily pushed her and then left the house. He returned less than an hour later to find his wife dead and a house full of police. In his momentary "loss of control" he had pushed his wife through a plate-glass window, and she bled to death on the front lawn while her husband "walked off his anger." I detached the card with phone numbers and safety plans from the brochure, somewhere in my heart recognizing that I, too, was in danger of being "accidentally" pushed down a flight of stairs or through a window.

Many years later, I would send community-education volunteers and staff to sit in booths at malls and street fairs. When they returned, they often complained that no one really stopped to talk to them. "But did they walk away with materials?" I asked, and the answer was invariably yes. I told them about my carrying a card for years before I actually used it. "You may never know firsthand about the difference you made today. There are thousands of women like me who carry a card in their wallet or write down a phone number from a poster tacked to the back of the door in a women's restroom. You may well have helped to save someone's life today, and you will never know it."

I was lucky: I lived in a town with a shelter, the shelter had space available, and my call wasn't left on an answering machine or routed through an answering service. A real person answered my call, a person who had authority to give me directions and tell me to come in.

At that time shelters were just beginning to emerge across the nation, but Wyoming was already committed to ensuring that a network of regional shelter programs was available to assist women and children in danger. Part of the reason for that was, in Wyoming, if you have no home to go to, you may very well end up frozen on the side of the road. The vast, frozen, windswept deserts can be brutal and unforgiving. Laramie is built on a high mountain plateau surrounded by peaks, many covered with snow year round. Once the snow starts falling in early autumn, the ground will be blanketed until late spring. Growing up in Kansas, I was familiar with the small wooden fences that are built to protect roads from blowing snow. But Wyoming highways are bordered by enormous snow walls, stacked one atop another up the sides of mountains.

The SAFE Project maintained its shelter in a confidential location, like most do. I was directed to a large house near the University of Wyoming and told to park in the back, where my car would be out of sight. Like every shelter I have been in since, the ramshackle house was filled with a mish-mash of well-worn, donated furniture and goods. A kitchen table ringed by folding chairs served as the client-intake and group-gathering spot.

After providing minimal information, my two sons and I were assigned a bedroom with one full-size bed where I slept with two-year-old Cody. Brandon, still a baby, got a crib. At no point did I ever have to prove my allegations of abuse. For the first time, I was believed without question. Because I came directly from work and had been warned against going to my home, I brought nothing for any of us except the clothes we wore. The staff provided diapers for Brandon, toothbrushes and toothpaste, shampoo and soap, nightclothes, and a change of clothes for the next day. We were also given food and the chance to talk.

I was still deep in denial and horribly embarrassed that I, a social-service professional in a small community, was asking for help from a partner agency. SAFE Project's executive director was a friend and a peer; I had even served on the board for a short while. I was also the only woman in the shelter that day who was well educated and held a professional job. So I kept to myself, rebuffing all attempts by fellow residents and staff to reach out to me. I think I believed I was above this whole mess or in some way better than the others. I was wrong.

During the five years of my marriage, and even since the divorce, I had fled my home on occasions too numerous to count. I was one of the many battered women who, when things got difficult, pulled out my credit card and ran to a hotel. I avoided the perceived embarrassment of a shelter, thinking my situation wasn't bad enough to justify taking up space. I thought I could handle the crisis, or I could just stay away until Jay calmed down. On more than one occasion I had driven across the country to my family, or spent the night, pregnant and with a small child, behind two locked doors on my office floor. But most often I ran to my friend Morita's home. Her two little boys were the same ages as mine, and she and her husband always welcomed me until it felt safe for us to return to our own house.

I stayed at the shelter for only three days because Jay entered an inpatient drug-and-alcohol-treatment program located in another state. He had agreed to the treatment program to lessen a jail sentence handed down when he got into a drunken brawl. His counselor in Laramie, a recovering alcoholic himself, arranged for him to attend a pro-bono program in Kansas. Jay's leaving the state enabled me to move back home and experience several weeks of peace.

More important, despite my aloofness and denial, my three days at the shelter allowed me to begin to connect with other women experiencing abuse, and to recognize that what I was experiencing wasn't normal. That old kitchen table with its folding chairs became a lifeline. I began to see that, just possibly, I was not alone. I also began to truly understand that maybe the abuse wasn't my fault.

How had I ever reached a point where I hid from my ex-husband, thinking his kicks and punches, his threats and intimidation, could be my fault? Despite years of soul-searching, I'm not sure I know the answer yet. I've looked back at my life many times, trying to find clues. Before I met Jay, I had two long-time boyfriends, neither of them violent. Randy was a high school baseball player, and Jorge was a real-live Spanish count studying in the United States. I am now happily married. Clearly, I wasn't just drawn to abusive men or in some way compelled to be a "victim." I talk to women all the time who say, "I would never put up with that. The first time and I would have been out of there." I have learned that such choices are rarely so straightforward. Had the abuse started with a direct kick or a punch I probably would have been out of there too, but battering is much more than the physical abuse and the withering assaults on my self-esteem that seemed designed to crush my soul. Perhaps, as you read my story, you will discern some "psychological defect" that doomed me to this brief but catastrophic marriage. But I think not.

I was the second of five children, born in Dodge City, Kansas, to Jack and Melva White. My parents were both in their teens when they married, and they promptly birthed five children in as many years. "All I have to do is walk by the bedroom door and throw in my dirty underwear, and she comes out pregnant," my father used to joke. In many ways, Dodge City was an idyllic community in which to be young. We could walk and ride our bikes almost anywhere in town, and someone always knew one of our parents, grandmothers, aunts, uncles, or cousins. At age three I was allowed to walk the two blocks to my grandmother's house with my older sister, Jacque. The town was famous for its history as the wickedest little town in the West, a reputation earned when Texas cattlemen drove their longhorns north to the railroad's end. The cowboys spent their paychecks on prostitutes and liquor, sometimes ending up buried in Boot Hill — with their boots on — after a gunfight. By the time I came along, though, the cowboys and prostitutes were all gone. Sturdy German farmers took their place, people with the skills to farm the wind-scoured prairies.

We were poor, but I didn't know it. We lived in a big old farmhouse at the edge of town, complete with an ancient combine behind the barn. No one can imagine a better jungle gym. Our favorite playground was packed dirt at the back of the yard, shaded by a giant cottonwood whose spreading limbs welcomed children intent on playing house. Each limb was a separate room. We also roamed the nearby fields of corn, playing hide-and-seek among the stalks. My memories of those days shimmer with the joys of playing outside and spending time with our extended clan. However, I also remember being plagued by night terrors and the realization that all was not calm on the home front. My young father barely earned a living as a traveling salesman for the Sunshine Biscuit Co., and sometimes he didn't come home as scheduled. My mother often ran out of money, and we filled ourselves on biscuits and gravy for supper and milk toast for breakfast. As an adult I was told that only poor families ate milk toast. I had always considered it a special treat.

When I was in second or third grade my parents moved the entire family to Wichita, the biggest city in Kansas, in order to gain access to better schools for my sister and me. Leaving her family was hard on my mother, so we made the three-hour drive to Dodge City almost every weekend. Still, the move was deemed successful when Jacque and I were tested and invited to attend the public school in Wichita for "accelerated students." I look back in awe that my mother and father, still practically kids themselves, moved their family of seven away from everything they knew just to provide educational opportunity for their two little girls. My father, the most widely read person I ever met, never achieved more than a high school diploma. Largely self-educated, his knowledge of history was equivalent to that of someone with a PhD. My mother, also an avid reader, didn't even finish high school. I was blessed to be brought up in a house full of books: all of the great classics, plus volumes on history, geography, art, travel, geology, and archeology. Both of my parents valued education so much that every one of their five children graduated from college. Because of their thorough indoctrination, I didn't fully realize that attending college was a choice until I had almost finished.

I graduated from high school in Wichita. Although chubby as a child, as a teenager I grew to a height of five-foot-ten. I ran with the popular crowd, but I was often desperately unhappy. I am embarrassed to admit that I felt humiliated by my family's circumstances, by the banged-up old car my mother drove and my family's continuing financial difficulties. Like many teens, I think I cared too much about appearances. I started babysitting at age thirteen, thereafter buying my own clothes and trying to pay my own way. But my father had again started staying away for days and weeks at a time, and my mother was often left alone with five children, trying to dodge the calls of irate bill collectors. I felt as though I lived two different lives: the smart and vibrant girl at school and the scared kid at home. And I certainly learned how to keep secrets, how to pretend that everything was fine when things were really coming apart. I was a people pleaser, desperate to fit in, and I never felt as though I really belonged anywhere.

My family moved back to western Kansas after I graduated from high school, settling in Coldwater, a no-stoplight town of about 700 residents. My parents gave me many gifts, and being born and reared in western Kansas was one of the best. Described in the 1800s as the "Great American Desert," it is big land with horizons and skies that seem to go on forever. I learned about the cycles of planting and harvest. In the weeks approaching wheat harvest, entire communities wait for the crops to ripen, praying that hail and thunderstorms won't destroy an entire year's hard work. In the final days before the harvest, the wheat fields look like undulating oceans of gold.

I learned about self-sufficiency, while also counting on neighbors, family, and friends when one needs a "hand up." I learned that you don't give up. Life can be tough, but you work hard, believe in family, and play the hand you're dealt. I learned that as a female in a man's world, I should always be able to take care of myself and not count on anyone else to provide me with a secure life. Yet, somehow, I also came to believe that as a woman my life wouldn't be complete unless I had a man to care about me.

I attended the University of Kansas in Lawrence, a long way, both geographically and culturally, from the western plains. I often worked full-time as a waitress, taking evening and weekend shifts so I could attend a full load of classes during weekdays. The schedule significantly limited my social life. During my junior year I was hired to wait tables at the Lawrence Country Club, where I made an automatic 15 percent gratuity. As far as I was concerned, I was in "fat city." I actually had to take a cut in pay when I graduated and accepted a professional position in a nonprofit agency. However, working at the country club also reinforced my persistent sense of inferiority. I remember the evening after a football game when many of the girlfriends I had gone to high school with came in to eat with other members of their sorority. I, of course, could never take off work to attend the games because they were some of our busiest days, let alone incur the extra expense of joining a sorority, and now I had to serve my former friends. The gulf between their lives and mine seemed immense, and it felt like they had won the lottery in life.

I dated my high-school boyfriend, Randy, through most of college until I met Jorge, the Spanish count, during my senior year. Jorge lived in an apartment across the hall from me. He was funny and charming and adored me. I was crazy about him as well, and I thought we would marry. However, while on a much-anticipated and saved-for college graduation trip to visit Jorge's family in Spain, it became clear to me that I couldn't marry him and move to Barcelona and live the affluent and spoiled lifestyle he promised. My nascent feminist philosophies were roused when I observed how fundamentally different the role of a woman was in Spanish culture. Jorge assured me that he would "allow" me to do anything I wanted. The word "allow" wasn't something I could get past. So in 1975, after graduating with a degree in occupational therapy, I bade Jorge farewell and accepted a job in Colby, a town of five thousand located in far northwestern Kansas.

Colby's primary economy centers on ranching, farming, and interstate travel to and from the distant Colorado mountains. Most people know it as a string of featureless motels, truck stops, and fast-food outlets scattered along two highway exits marking the flat, endless prairie. I was hired as the program coordinator for a regional nonprofit organization providing therapeutic and educational services for children with physical and developmental disabilities. It was a much more important job than I could ever have landed as a new graduate in a larger city, and it afforded me multiple opportunities for professional growth. However, I failed to factor in the impact on my social life and the loneliness of living in a tiny town.

I was one of only a handful of young, single, professional people living and working in Colby. On most weekends I drove two hours south to Coldwater. On some weeknights I ventured out with friends from work to Colby's main hotspot, a bar and dance club called the Rusty Bucket.

I first met Jay at the Rusty Bucket. He was one of the handsomest men I had ever met, like a tall, dark version of a young Mel Gibson, and he looked completely out of place in a bar full of farmers, custom cutters, and oil field workers. We danced and talked, and I gave him my phone number. Jay called the next day, we talked some more, and he asked if I would like to go out with him that evening. I fibbed and said I was busy. He then asked me out for the following weekend. I agreed, but with some trepidation.

Jay, who was one year younger than I, was smart — he had skipped several grades in school — and he was charming. He said he was in the middle of a divorce and was living in his parent's basement in Colby while trying to get his life together. He didn't seem to have a job, and he had an arrogance and glib charm that I found disturbing. I was never much of a casual dater, and as the weekend approached I realized I didn't really want to pursue a relationship with this man. I told him I had to go out of town and couldn't make it after all.

That weekend I decided against driving down to Coldwater and stayed in town with Billy, my beloved toy Peke-a-poo. On Saturday, while I sat on my front porch throwing a ball for Billy, feeling lonely and questioning what I was doing living by myself in this remote corner of Kansas, Jay cruised past my house in his big white car. Another man might have been embarrassed to catch someone in such an obvious lie, but Jay just rolled down his window as he drove slowly past, waving nonchalantly.

Never one to be deterred, he drove by again about thirty minutes later. This time he stopped and came over to join me on the porch to play with Billy. Put so obviously on the spot, I again fibbed and said I decided at the last minute against going out of town. He just laughed, making it clear he knew I was embarrassed about not being truthful with him.

I know now that Jay's "drive-bys," which foreshadowed his later stalking, should have been a huge red flag. But he made me feel special, and he befriended my best friend, my dog Billy. I was fearful of where I was going with my life. What kind of future could I ever hope to build in Colby, Kansas? Always a "fixer," I soon decided this was a man with potential, and he just needed a good woman. I saw no signs of his future violence, and I wasn't put off by his lack of a job. He just needed to find himself, I thought; after all, my own father got a very slow start in creating a viable career.

Jay didn't start out hurting me. He courted me and made me feel desirable. We began an intensely passionate relationship, and he truly made me feel he couldn't live without me. He constantly showered me with flowers and gifts, and with his attentions. He worked sporadically doing construction, and most of his meager earnings went toward wooing me.

I believed that Jay needed me to help him get through his divorce, find a career, and deal with the imminent death of his father from lung cancer. He just needed me to help him be whole. His family also perceived me as his salvation, the woman who was helping their brilliant but troubled son and brother to pull his life together. His family embraced me at a desperately lonely time in my life.

Looking back, I realize we moved too fast. We were married in six months, because Jay and his entire family were adamant that we needed to marry before his father died. He wanted his father to die in peace, believing his troubled son had found his way. Always a people-pleaser, I wanted his family to be happy.

From the very beginning, Jay was surprisingly overpossessive. I first caught glimpses of his abuse during jealous tantrums, which usually were associated with some imagined flirtation on my part. I think I may have been flattered that he cared so intensely. I did not suspect that these tantrums would grow into full-blown rages after our marriage. I wish I had recognized the warning signs of a very damaged young man who, despite what he assured me and what I believed, would not be able to change.

One particular incident before our marriage was pretty horrific. Because Jay didn't have a college degree or a viable career, it was clear to me that others who had more education and professional success intimidated him. My boss, Jim, whom I held in high regard, fit those criteria. Jim, a devoted husband and father, was a former Catholic monk who truly lived the values of humility, integrity, and honor. I considered him a friend and a mentor, which brought out Jay's demons in a very public and humiliating way. Jay and I attended a holiday party for staff and family associated with my job. It was the first and only time in my life that I won the door prize, a holiday ham, and I was having a great time with all of the people from work. I completely lost track of Jay and assumed he was having a good time as well, hanging out with others in a different room.

As it turned out, he was in the back room drinking to the point of being sloppy and argumentative. Jim, seeing what was happening, attempted to calm Jay and move him away from the alcohol. With no provocation other than a kind word from Jim, Jay erupted into a whirlwind of biting, kicking, punching, screaming, and name-calling. Before I even knew what was going on the police had been called and Jay was being transported to the jail, where he spent the night in a padded cell, restrained in a strait jacket.

Afterwards, Jay blamed his actions on the alcohol. Also, Jim said he wouldn't come to our wedding because he didn't want to cause any embarrassment for Jay. I was humiliated, and everyone else was embarrassed and tried to act as though nothing had happened. Nothing further was said.

How in the world — you want to know — could I go ahead and marry this man? The short answer is, clearly, flawed judgment. I was very good at denying what I didn't want to deal with. My judgment was also clouded by the fact that Jay's father was dying from cancer, and his entire family had vested enormous hope in our marriage. Domestic violence wasn't widely known about or talked about and was still considered by most to be a private family matter. And I was naïve about alcohol. Everyone in college drank to excess, and I thought Jay's actions were the result of his drunkenness. I didn't know Jay to be much of a drinker, so I hoped this incident was an anomaly. Only much later did I begin to realize I had actually spent my entire life around gentle drunks, their drinking neither acknowledged nor spoken about.

After our short engagement, we were married in a small ceremony in Colby, attended by family and a few friends. Jay's father died a month later. Then, slowly at first, Jay's rage began to focus on me. The first time he raised a hand to me was when I returned from a trip to Lawrence for a training program. While in town, I stopped by Jorge's apartment to get the big rubber tree he had been keeping for me since my move out West. Jay got home after I did, and he stormed in screaming at me as I sat on the couch in our living room waiting for him to help me carry the rubber tree into the house. He was frenzied, accusing me of imagined indiscretions with my former boyfriend, screaming about what I must have done to convince him to give me back the rubber tree. Raging, Jay upended the couch where I sat, leaving me tumbled in a heap with the furniture on top of me.

I was astonished. I'd never tried to hide the visit to Jorge, because in my mind, and in reality, the visit was perfectly innocent. My tumble didn't hurt me, but Jay's response and actions terrified me. However, I bought into his insistence that I had provoked the attack by seeing an old boyfriend. I knew how jealous he was; I should never have stopped to get my rubber plant. It was my fault this had happened.

I think this is one of the most difficult things for people to understand about battered women. One's thinking begins to change to accommodate the reality around them. And thus began an odyssey all too familiar to battered women. If I just said the right things, wore my hair right, dressed right, talked to the right people, didn't talk to the wrong people, cooked the right thing for dinner, had sex when and how he wanted it, came home from work on time, answered the phone when he called, and read his mind in every possible respect, I thought I could make things okay. I worked very hard to control Jay's alcohol intake; his violent rages were most unpredictable when he drank.

I was committed to the marriage, as I thought I should be. I was convinced things would improve if only Jay were happier and more self-assured. We tried a geographic fix, moving hundreds of miles northwest to Casper, Wyoming. Like many battered women before and after me, I thought life would be easier if we went someplace where we could both start with a clean slate. Since I was an occupational therapist, it was pretty easy for me to find good jobs that paid fairly well. I also thought it would be wise to move farther from my family, whom Jay hated, and vice-versa. When he was with them, he quickly started feeling threatened and became overbearing, so I tried to keep them apart. Because my own relationship with my mother had often been contentious, Jay sometimes convinced me his response was justified. Now, however, I know that isolation from family and friends is another red flag.

I rarely visited home, and my family came to see us even more infrequently, but one time my mother and brother Steve came to visit us in Casper. Earlier that week Jay had hurled a handful of coins at me, leaving small crescent-shaped bruises all over my face. When she saw me, my mother became quite upset, immediately suspecting that Jay had been hurting me. I don't remember what justification I gave, but I was becoming pretty adept at making excuses.

The visit went quickly downhill; within hours my mother, always somewhat volatile, and Jay were screaming at each other. My gangly, six-foot-eight brother, also known for his unpredictable temper, intervened on my mother's side. Jay sprang across the room toward Steve. My mother stepped between them, and Jay slugged her while trying to get at my brother.

Yes, my husband had now physically assaulted my mother—but, as I desperately tried to rationalize, he wasn't trying to hit her; he was trying to hit my brother. And my brother had always been able to make us all unreasonably angry. It was a horrible incident, but through my convoluted thinking I could see how it had happened. Surely 100 percent of the blame wasn't with Jay, was it?

Completely enraged, and certain that their prior estimation of Jay was now confirmed, my mother and brother left for home, taking only a few moments to fling their suitcases and clothing into the back of the car. Devastated by the events, I made Jay move out of the house that very day, and within the week I rented the main floor of our house to a small family and moved to the basement, counting on the additional income to help me cover the house payments. I knew I couldn't look to Jay to provide any support once he was out of the house.

Within a few days my slow-to-anger father wrote me saying that as long as I was married to Jay I was "no longer his daughter." I still vividly remember sitting in the tiny bath of the basement I now called home, reading the pages written in my father's cramped, barely legible hand. My father had always been my best friend and advocate, and I was truly devastated by the letter and the level of anger directed at me. I couldn't believe how unfair it felt that he sent the letter without even speaking with me first. I was now completely isolated, alienated from my family, living in a place where I had many acquaintances but no real friends or allies. I had learned to keep my secrets well, and keeping my secrets meant keeping others at arm's length. If I let anyone close, I might have to explain things I couldn't even understand myself.

After only a couple of years of marriage, and now living separately, Jay and I started counseling. As with many marriage counselors then and now, the therapist totally failed to recognize or acknowledge the abuse that was destroying our marriage. He ignored the physical and emotional danger to me. Instead, he focused on how to make Jay feel better about himself and what I could and should do to help with the process. My parents were married more than fifty years, and I took to heart "for better for worse, in sickness and in health," because their marriage had certainly not been easy. I thought I was doing the right thing in standing by Jay, and I thought I still loved him. I still believed I could help him heal from the pain and anger he carried inside. Looking back, I think perhaps I had somehow learned to forgive too much. I wonder sometimes if I knew then what real love even looked like.

Eventually, with the support of the marriage counselor, we reconciled and decided to move to Laramie, three hours south, so Jay could enter the University of Wyoming. My role was to provide encouragement and financial support; I thought that if Jay could get a degree and come to feel better about himself, our lives could be more peaceful, a belief our counselor encouraged. Nevertheless, our marriage continued to deteriorate rapidly. I took a lower-paying job to facilitate a move to Laramie, where Jay enrolled as a freshman at the university. He had always worked only sporadically and now declared that he needed to devote himself full-time to his studies. Still trying to be the supportive wife, I accepted this decision even though I had worked full-time to put myself through college and we were struggling financially, which was further stressing the marriage.

Within weeks of our move, I discovered I was pregnant. Although the pregnancy wasn't planned, we were both delighted with the news. I loved everything about being pregnant: the feeling of my baby growing inside me, the changes in my body, the little flutter kicks, and even the elbows under my ribs. What I didn't love or expect was Jay's reaction to my progressing pregnancy. While I bonded with the perfect little person I carried, Jay spent his time hanging out with friends from school, drinking beer and endlessly smoking marijuana. His friends were mostly first-year students like himself, but they were eighteen and nineteen years old and didn't have wives and families. Jay was fully embracing the student experience with little thought for the responsibilities associated with his growing family.

When he did come home, we argued about money, his drinking, and his pot smoking. Most arguments deteriorated into Jay's throwing things against walls, kicking holes in doors, verbally threatening me, and occasionally throwing objects at me. Still, I felt I had even more reason to "try to make our marriage work." I was convinced our child needed a father. Jay continued to work at his studies, and he controlled his rages much better than he had in the past. The kicks and punches were rarely aimed in my direction. After every rampage, Jay apologized profusely, telling me he couldn't live without me and was trying hard to become a better person.

I worked until the day before I delivered my son. Since we only had one car, I usually walked to and from work. Three weeks from my due date, I was walking home when I realized I just couldn't make it, so I plopped down on a curb about three blocks from our house. Jay eventually realized that I seemed to be taking longer then usual and came looking for me in the car. That night I went into labor, and Cody was born early the next morning. My job didn't allow for maternity leave, so I went back to work two weeks after delivering, and Jay cared for Cody until he was six weeks old and could be enrolled in day care. In a stroke of good luck, I was hired within a few months of Cody's birth to run an agency that was located in the same building as Cody's day care, thus dramatically lessening my daily stress level.

I continued to be fully invested in Jay's having time for his "studies," not knowing that Jay had quit attending classes. He was spending his days at the student union playing chess, or off-campus getting high with his friends. It wasn't until many months later that I discovered his ruse. This was the absolute last straw for me. I asked him to leave, and I found a divorce attorney. Money was tight, but I had a decent job and knew I would be better off on my own. He moved in with a friend from school, but he called incessantly and came by the house daily without any notice.

There were several stops and starts in the course of our separation and divorce. My parents and I were now speaking, but I was still quite isolated from my family and was often quite lonely. After several months, Jay and I reconciled for a week. We then separated again, and I continued to pursue a divorce, which was harder than it sounds due to our desperate financial situation. I certainly had no money to pay an attorney.

A month after the reconciliation, I discovered I was pregnant with our second child. I had gone into work early one morning because I was driving to Jackson Hole with some colleagues. I felt kind of queasy, and someone joked, "Maybe it's morning sickness." My life crashed down around me in that moment. Of course it was morning sickness. I had a one-year old, I was divorcing an abusive husband, and I was pregnant. I remember sitting in the back seat of the car on the seven-hour drive, replaying my life in my head, wondering how I was going to do this.

Then things really got crazy. The most dangerous point in an abusive relationship is when a woman tries to leave. In textbook fashion, as Jay recognized that he was losing me, he escalated the abuse. I admit to being a part of the craziness. Although Jay was tracking my every move, he also had relationships with other women and, feeling unattractive and a failure as a wife and a lover, I spiraled into despair. I had trouble sleeping, eating, and managing the realities of my job while caring for the baby I carried inside of me as well as one-year-old Cody. This is the part of my history with Jay that is most fuzzy in my memory, no doubt because of the increasing abuse, the emotional stress, and the changing hormones caused by my pregnancy. My strongest memories from this time are not of events but of emotional impressions of incredible pain and grief. I remember sitting on the floor of my bathroom, the room most distant from my sleeping baby, wedged between the toilet and the shower, doubled over, wailing so loud and with such sorrow that I didn't know how I could possibly survive the pain.

Because of my pregnancy, Jay and I tried a second reconciliation, but he continued a relationship with another woman. He denied having any involvements, but his protestations were weak. I eventually confronted the other woman with my suspicions. She said he told her we didn't sleep together and had no marriage except in name only. She said he wore no wedding ring when he was with her.

How, I wondered, could this man who lived a life in total disarray, who couldn't remember to pick up his son at day care at the same time every day, manage an illicit affair while maintaining a charade of marriage? How could he possibly remember to take off and put on his wedding ring on cue?

We separated once again, and I continued with divorce proceedings. Daily, Jay called me twenty to thirty times and drove by my house eight or ten times. I took to staying home when not at work so I would be there for his calls and not risk escalating his behavior. He worked erratically, which gave him time to carefully monitor my comings and goings. Whenever he came by the house, his visits deteriorated into verbal and physical attacks. I suspected then, and know now, that my craziness was in continuing to allow this man into my home and my life. I thought that I owed him as the father of my children, that I still loved him, and that I was the only one who could help him to find himself. I insanely believed him when he said that I "made him do these things."

One night I told Jay I was absolutely proceeding with the divorce. He didn't erupt as I expected; instead, he left me alone in the family room and went to another part of the house. I thought the time-out seemed like a good idea. But he returned a few minutes later, a large envelope in his hand.

"I will show you exactly what you can do with this marriage," he said. He took our marriage license from the envelope, tore it into several large pieces, and held me down while he stuffed the parchment down my throat. I truly thought this was the moment I would die. I was choking on the paper and, with Jay sitting on my chest, I couldn't breathe. I was cold with terror as I struggled for breath. Cody was screaming, which eventually seemed to bring his father back to his senses. Jay let me up so I could pull the paper from my throat. He then slammed out of the house, leaving me huddled on the floor with Cody in my arms.

Jay continued to control my every move and treat me as a possession. My response was to work hard to maintain the peace. I didn't have the options available to me that many women have today; no laws were in place to protect battered women, and even divorced women were perceived as their ex-husband's property. I remember a counselor telling me that the best way to get Jay to leave me alone would be for me to marry another man. In Jay's eyes, I would then become that man's possession, and Jay could no longer assert his ownership.

As crazy as it sounds, I have difficulty stating exactly at what point we were finally divorced. Getting divorced, like everything else in my marriage, was harder than it needed to be. I told my attorney, a kindly man who agreed to let me pay his fees over time, to do whatever needed to be done to get me out of the marriage. I had only two conditions: custody of my children and possession of the washer and dryer. Any mother can tell you the two go together. "Don't put any child support into the decree because it will just be a point for dissension," I told him. He said the judge simply would not allow that to go through, so instead he requested the absolute minimum.

Jay refused to acknowledge the process in any way. When served with papers he wouldn't take them, when asked to negotiate he didn't return phone calls, and when asked to sign documents he tore them up. Eventually, the divorce was given by decree because of Jay's total non-compliance. We had been married for five years.

Things were so difficult with Jay during this period that I was fearful to have my mother come to help me when the baby arrived, even though I desperately needed her help because I was living alone, working full-time, and already had a small child. I knew I couldn't count on Jay for help, but I also knew my family's presence enraged him. I just wanted to try to maintain the status quo, to have peace in my little corner of the world at any price. If my mother or any other family member came, I instinctively knew Jay would perceive it as a further loss of control, and his behavior would escalate. A friend took care of Cody, just two years old, when I went into the hospital to give birth to Brandon. I came home after only a day, but Brandon was jaundiced and had to stay in the hospital for several more days. I took Cody with me to the hospital every three hours to breastfeed Brandon until I could take him home with me.

Hospital personnel knew that something was terribly wrong in my life. Bruises marred my face and forehead when I went into labor, and despite being eight-and-a-half months pregnant I was almost gaunt. My pediatrician came to talk to me after Brandon's birth, prompted, I think, by the nurses to ask me about the bruises on my face. I brushed my hair across my forehead and told him I was "okay." By that time I was so tired and overwhelmed that I didn't even bother to try to make up an excuse. My saying I was okay seemed to be all the assurance he needed, and the subject was dropped.

The nurses, clearly dismayed, tried speaking with me about my home arrangements; I was going home with a newborn and a two-year-old without any support at all. My friend Morita, the one person to whom I always turned, had just given birth herself. I couldn't in good conscience impose on her, and there was no one else. I realized how total my isolation was. Yet I seemed to have made it through the worst; I had given birth, and I was divorced. Things should have started getting better, but they didn't. Jay continued to control my every move through threats and what I have come to call domestic terrorism. I never had any idea when or where or what would provoke an outburst or attack. In addition, Brandon was born with serious asthma that often turned into pneumonia, and he was constantly in and out of the hospital.

I was now trying to work full-time and take care of a two-year-old and a seriously ill infant. Jay was the only person I could occasionally get to help me with Cody while I spent time with Brandon in the hospital. When Brandon was about six months old, he was referred to a specialist in Denver who placed him on a strict regimen of five or six medications, including a breathing treatment from a nebulizer every three hours. Each treatment took twenty minutes to administer. I remember driving home from Denver late on a Saturday afternoon, feeling complete despair. How in the world could I possibly handle his medication schedule by myself? On Monday morning I woke up and simply — began. I continued these treatments over the next eighteen months until Brandon was two years old and his asthma was better controlled.

I desperately needed Jay's assistance, and he was there for me sometimes. When I fell and broke my ankle playing softball with a group from work, I came home from the emergency room and sat on Brandon's bedroom floor as he cried in his crib and rambunctious Cody ran through the house. I couldn't drive and couldn't walk without crutches. The kitchen was on a different floor, and I couldn't figure out how to get Brandon, an infant, up the stairs to the main floor. Jay came by the house at that moment, and I would have let Frankenstein's monster in the door if he would just have helped me. Jay helped.

But every bit of help I got came at a hefty price. We were no longer married, but I was still Jay's property. When I tried to go out on a date, Jay kicked in the door to my house. When a male friend from high school visited, a former professional football player who slept on my family-room couch, I received anonymous, threatening, disgusting, and lewd phone calls for the two days he was there. Jay's voice was barely disguised on the other end of the line. When Jay's therapist called to tell me Jay was looking through my windows at night, fantasizing about shooting me as I slept, I began sleeping on my bedroom floor. I feared Cody would climb into my bed in the night and be shot instead. The therapist felt an obligation to warn me, but neither of us thought of telling the police. Jay hadn't actually done anything yet, and there were no stalking laws on the books at that time.

Despite everything that had gone on, and the general knowledge in the community about the ongoing harassment and abuse, I didn't look to the police for help. I thought the police would blame me or think I had provoked the attacks. That changed the day Jay came to pick up the boys for visitation and instead came into the house, to my bedroom, where he proceeded to rant and rave. He threatened me with a knife, which he used on my waterbed. Then he attacked me as I held our baby. Jay held the knife to my torso, eventually putting the weapon down to hit me with his fists. By the time he left, the room was destroyed, I was bruised and battered, and my little boys were traumatized. I called the police.

A young officer came to take my report. I showed him the bedroom and my emerging bruises. His primary questions were about the state of our relationship. Once he discerned that Jay was my ex-husband, he clearly lost interest. A couple of days later I had a meeting at work and the county attorney, a friend and board member, saw my bruises. She asked if I had called the police. I said I had, and she left to check on the status of the case. To her dismay and mine, there was no case. The responding officer had made no written report. "It was just a husband–wife thing," she was told when she tracked down the officer.

"You'd better write that report immediately and then arrest Jay and put his butt in jail," the county attorney told him. The most startling aspect of this incident, for me, was knowing that the only reason the system worked was because I knew the right people, people who could make it work. What if I had been poor, uneducated, or a member of an ethnic minority who already distrusted the system? What if I had been almost anyone else?

As a part of the subsequent court proceedings I was asked to detail the history of our marriage and Jay's ongoing abusive behavior. I finally, for the first time ever, told the whole story with all of the gory details. The judge read the written report and then spoke directly to Jay. "You are a walking time bomb, and when you go off, you are going to take this woman with you."

Rather than being frightened, I finally felt validated. I was not making this up or making it out to be worse than it was. The judge also said he was sorry he could not afford me more protection, but, unfortunately, the arrest had been made as a probation violation for an earlier assault in a barroom fight, rather than for the assaults on me. It had apparently been more expedient to revoke probation than to file new charges. The most he could do, the judge stated, was to make Jay serve out the remainder of his earlier sentence. He went to jail after receiving a reduced sentence because he agreed to enter an alcohol-treatment program.

Jay's fury was inflamed by my breaking the bonds of silence. "Why did you tell them all of that stuff?" he asked me when he walked out of the courtroom.

"But it's all true," I said.

"I still can't believe you told them," he said.

Battering has flourished behind closed doors for centuries precisely because victims are reluctant to speak out, to shine a light into the dark corners and tell what is happening in supposedly loving homes. Twenty-five years ago, when I was living through these experiences, battering went largely unnoticed and unaddressed.

Another time, after the divorce, Jay gave me a painful black eye and bruised cheek, with multiple bruises and abrasions on the rest of my body. I left with my sons to drive to Colby to stay for a few days with Jay's mother, with whom I was quite close. She was safe; my going to her never escalated Jay's rage against me. Driving through Nebraska I was entertaining the boys with a tape of children's songs, singing along at the top of my lungs. I looked in my rearview mirror to see a police car, lights flashing, close on my tail. When I stopped I was told I was speeding and would need to pay the fine on the spot. I told him that I didn't have enough cash and that I had no credit cards, yet another casualty of my divorce. Informing me that he could not accept a check, the officer said he would have to take me to jail.

I followed him to the courthouse in a small rural town, where he threatened to jail me separately from my sons. I pointed out that I was still nursing the infant, so he relented and instead kept me sitting for the whole day while they called in a county judge from his farm so he could decide what to do with me, an apparently hardened criminal, covered with bruises, speeding down a Nebraska highway singing children's songs with my two little boys. They finally allowed me to write a personal check to pay the exorbitant fine and to go on my way. At no point did any of the officers of the court ask me about my black eye and bruises, turning a willfully oblivious eye to my condition.

I distinctly remember the moment at which I fully recognized that the abuse wasn't my fault and my actions weren't what was making Jay lose control. Despite the physical and emotional pain, the alienation from my own family, the arrest and the judge's statement, I had continued, at some level, to buy into Jay's assertions that I made him do these things. The years of physical, emotional, and verbal assaults had taken their toll on my self-confidence and belief in my own judgment. My final moment of enlightenment was triggered by a relatively minor event. I had been to the store and had a sack of groceries in the front seat, with Cody and Brandon buckled into their car seats in the back. I saw Jay walking down the street and offered him a ride to his apartment. He hopped in the car, moving the groceries from the seat to the floor. When I stopped in front of his apartment, he talked to the boys for a minute, then turned to rifle through the groceries. The next thing I knew he had shoved a pint of sour cream into my face, splattering everything in the car. Sour cream was on the rearview mirror, in the console, on the dash, in my ears and nostrils — absolutely everywhere.

"Why?" I stammered in total shock as I wiped sour cream from the inside of my sunglasses.

"You only buy sour cream when you're having someone over for dinner," he snarled.

Jay's logic confounded me. Yes, I often made a special dish for company using sour cream. No, I wasn't planning on having any guests for dinner. And finally, even if I were having guests over, what would be wrong with that? This was a turning point for me. His hold over me was broken.

As Jay's control over me deteriorated, he became even more frantic to maintain it. When threats against me didn't work, he threatened to take the boys. When that didn't work, he threatened suicide. And when that didn't work, he told me he was dying of a brain tumor. Of course, he wasn't. When asked years later if I ever thought about killing Jay, I could honestly answer no. But at some point I did begin to wish that he would follow through on his threats to kill himself.

I began to see that if I continued to live in Laramie, I would never be free of Jay. Yet I was the sole support for two little boys, and I had a good job that I loved. I also had a house I couldn't sell. The real estate market in Laramie was deeply depressed, and I had tried selling my home but had no offers even when I listed it for less than what I paid. Most importantly, it felt unfair that I should be the one who had to leave. So I stayed and continued to try to manage the situation as best I could.

Despite the trauma and pain, in many ways this was a time of great joy. I was completely in love with my little boys. Brandon was a soft, smiling, curly-headed, roly-poly, lovebug of a child. Cody talked nonstop and climbed, jumped, and ran everywhere he went. As the older of the two, Cody was also becoming increasingly aware of what was going on, and his anxiety manifested through behavioral problems at home and day care.

The situation was complicated by my conflicted feelings; I no longer wanted Jay in my life, but I continued to hope he would be the kind of father my sons needed and deserved. Furthermore, even had I wanted to, I had no legal standing to keep him away from the boys. Jay paid no child support and regularly attacked their mom in front of them, but legally I had no right to keep him from seeing his sons.

Everything finally came falling down around my ears one Sunday in early March 1984, nearly two years after the attack that caused me to seek safety at the battered women's shelter. Jay was to take the boys for the day, and when he showed up at my house he seemed reasonable and happy. I invited him inside while I finished getting the boys ready for their outing. Jay asked for something to drink, so I directed him to the refrigerator. As I knelt in the family room to tie Brandon's shoes, I was suddenly ducking cans of beer as they came hurtling at my head. Within moments, my sons were crying, beer was flying, and I was diving for the phone. Apparently, a six pack of beer in my refrigerator was yet another indication of sexual indiscretion on my part.

Jay grabbed the phone from me and threw me across the room into the loveseat. The boys and I cowered together as Jay stomped back and forth before us, raging. By now, I saw only ugliness when I looked at what I had once considered a movie-star handsome face — a face that was distorted with rage and heavy with brutality and deceit, a face I had once adored but had grown to pity and even hate. I remember looking at that face and wondering how I had ever let this monster into my life.

One thing made this incident different from all the ones that had come before. Working himself into a frenzy, Jay grabbed me off the couch, but this time Cody jumped between us. Cody, my three-year-old son, was so attuned to my moods and thoughts that sometimes I believed he could read my mind. This son, deeply disturbed by the ongoing violence, turmoil, and his mother's anguish, put himself between his father and me in an effort to protect me.

What I would learn much later, after I began my work with battered women's programs, is that the most common reason a woman finally chooses to leave her batterer is because the violence has begun to be directed at the children.

Jay's violence wasn't actually directed at Cody; it was directed at me — and whoever got in the way. Cody wasn't really hurt that time. He had no cuts, scrapes, or bruises, but he was thrown crying across the room. I suddenly understood with great clarity what lay ahead for my sons if I were to continue to try to "manage" this horrific relationship between their father and me.

Jay eventually released me when a friend started calling repeatedly to check on me, knowing Jay was supposed to come by that morning to get the boys. When I didn't answer the phone, the friend kept calling until Jay finally answered, immediately prompting the friend to tell him she would be calling the police. He released us and left the house. As soon as he was gone, I picked up newspapers from Denver and Albuquerque, scouring the want ads. This time I knew I had to get us away from the insanity. I found a couple of possibilities and sent off resumes by the end of the day. The listing for the job in Denver was an ambiguous posting for an executive director. No agency was named, and the reply went to a post office box. The skills they were seeking seemed to fit well with my own: They asked for experience with grant writing, fund-raising, volunteer management, staff management, and working with boards.

I went to work the next day and told my board chair I was quitting and moving away. I called a realtor about putting my house on the market again and talked to my bank about the feasibility of signing a quitclaim deed, giving the property back to the bank. I had made up my mind. I was leaving. Sometimes, I decided, running away is the right and smart thing to do.

I later learned that the chair of the board called other board members, asking how they might convince me to change my mind and stay.

"She's doing the right thing," said the county attorney, who was still on the board. "The best thing we can do is to give her an armed escort to the state line and wish her well."

2

surviving
and
speaking out:
building my life
free from violence

You must see hundreds of women walk in and out of these doors. They come and they go, angry, bitter, frightened, and you touch each of their lives. Perhaps you think they won't remember you, but when you meet them, a seed is planted. It either grows in fertile soil, or it stays dormant until one day, maybe unknown to you, a new life peeks above the dirt to see the sun. So, dear friend, a tiny part of you is left in each woman, and they will never be the same.

—A shelter client

S EVERAL YEARS LATER, I SAT WITH MY MOTHER IN A FOOD court in a Denver mall and spoke, circumspectly and with a lot of apprehension, about some incident from my time with Jay. My mother, who never discussed the personal trials she experienced growing up poor in a single-parent home or during her years of raising five children as little more than a child herself, said, "I just hate it that this all happened to you. I really wish you had never gone through all of this."

Her statement, and her unexpected sentiment, gave me pause. If I had not endured those years with Jay, a mere six or seven years out of an entire lifetime, would I have had the courage to break out of my box? Would I have tried for more in my life? I realized the answer was no. I didn't think I would ever have figured out that I was capable of being more than the insecure girl who never believed she was quite good enough. My life was changed forever by an abusive marriage. Trite as it may sound, from adversity I learned lessons for a lifetime. I had been living in a box created by my own self-expectations, and I had no choice but to break out. I discovered I was more powerful, more competent, and more capable than I had ever dreamed. I found reservoirs of courage I could call upon to build a life for my children and myself. And I also learned how to help others recognize the same in themselves. I want to be very clear: I didn't come through the experience thinking I was special. But I did come through with total clarity on one important point: I was very lucky.

I regretted that my sons hadn't lived the idyllic lives I think most of us want for our children. In the best of all possible worlds, Jay would have conquered his demons and realized the potential we all believed lurked just below the surface of his chaotic, irrational behavior. He would have become the father my sons deserved and the husband I so desperately desired. But as hard as I tried, I simply couldn't make it so. My only viable choice was to run.

Leaving Laramie was no easy task, and I was terrified in a way I had never been while trying to manage things with Jay. What if I failed? Could I make it somewhere else alone with my boys? Moving home with my parents simply wasn't an option; tiny, isolated Coldwater held absolutely no opportunity for my little family. I had made the decision to leave, not knowing where I was going. Still, I began packing and making arrangements. I would have to create my own future.

A few days after I applied for jobs in other cities, I was eating dinner at my house with my friend Morita and our four little boys. The phone rang, a welcome distraction from our struggles to keep the food on the plates rather than ground into the carpets or thrown against the walls. When I answered, the woman on the other end of the line identified herself as the chair of the board of directors of Safehouse for Battered Women, located in Denver. Would I come for an interview?

Safehouse for Battered Women—the irony was astonishing. The blind ad to which I had responded the previous Sunday, after finally dislodging Jay from my home and calming my sons, was for the executive director of a battered women's shelter. Yes, I would come for an interview.

A week later I was on my way to Denver, nearly 150 miles south of Laramie across a mountain pass and through the foothills bordering the Rockies of Colorado and Wyoming. I later learned that more than two hundred people responded to the ad in the Denver newspaper. Nine went through the interview process, and I was offered the job. When I was asked during the interview whether I had ever been exposed to any domestic violence through my friends or family, I simply responded, "Yes."

My instincts told me that if I identified myself as a battered woman I would never be hired. I would be perceived as weak, flawed, and an inept manager. The disarray in my personal life would overshadow my years of success at running a nonprofit agency. Yet again, I would be the one blamed for what had happened. Much later, one of the directors involved in the interview told me my instincts were good. Had I elaborated on that answer, they never would have offered me the job.

As I said my goodbyes at the Developmental Preschool and Daycare, I sobbed uncontrollably. I doubted I would ever again love an organization and a job as I loved that agency. Every morning I brought my children with me to work, and I had the joy of watching them learn and grow, something most working mothers miss. I was also able to see children with seemingly crippling disabilities learn and grow in ways their parents had often been told were impossible.

Now I was taking a cut in pay to move to a large city where I didn't know a single soul. I had never before lived in a big city. I was a small-town girl, and cities, with their massive infrastructures, diversity, challenges, and opportunities, frightened me and inspired a weird kind of awe. When I was a senior in high school I took a trip with a group of friends to the Texas coast and saw the ocean for the first time; although Texans will tell you it is just the Gulf, to me it was definitely the ocean. Yet when I returned home and showed people the pictures I had taken, everyone was astonished to see that 90 percent were of the enormous highway interchanges I saw while traveling through Dallas and Houston. Yes, cities impressed me.

People asked what I would be doing in Denver, and at first I told them, but the moment I said the words "battered women's shelter," people's jaws would drop and I was met with disbelieving stares. I was embarrassed, convinced people might consider this a case of a lunatic running the asylum, so I started skipping over my answer or mumbling so quickly that people were left with just a vague impression. They knew I would be running something in Denver, but they weren't sure what. That was fine with me.

A young, no-nonsense student, Gillian Esson, had moved into my house at the semester break, just a couple of months before. We called her Gilly, and she helped me with the boys at night and on weekends. An internationally ranked racer with the University of Wyoming ski team, Gilly was often away for competitions. Nevertheless, she brought the first semblance of sanity to my life in what seemed like a very long time. I know that her assistance finally enabled me to pull myself together enough to move out of the state.

Gilly was fearless and tolerated absolutely no interference from Jay. By now, law enforcement officials paid attention when they received a call from my house, and she didn't hesitate to do whatever was necessary to protect my sons and me. Gilly has stayed my close friend to this day. Mercifully for her, she missed much of the strife that precipitated my move, but she saw and experienced enough to provide me with a reality check when I try to minimize what my life was like during that time. I have learned that battered women are great minimizers. If they truly acknowledge the extent of the turmoil and danger they endure, they might not be able to live with the pain.

My parents drove up from Kansas to help me with the move. They stayed at my house with me from the time I said I was leaving until the moment we pulled the U-Haul out of the driveway. Jay kept his distance. Friends and family surrounded me, forming a protective shield. On my last day in town Jay called my house in a despondent mood, telling me he had nothing left to live for.

"I'm sitting in my apartment with my gun in my mouth, and I'm going to kill myself," he said.

This time I believed him. On my way out of town I called the police and asked them to check on Jay, but I steadfastly drove toward the state line. Cody and Brandon, now almost two and four, were strapped into their car seats in the back of my trusty red Corolla. We headed toward our new lives. I felt as though I were making a great leap into the unknown.

Jay didn't kill himself that day, but I was finally free. He knew I had left to take a job at the Denver Safehouse for Battered Women; he had my phone number at work, but he had no other way to contact me. Safehouse operated from a confidential location, and I didn't tell him my new home address. His life had fallen into such a state of disarray that he didn't have the funds or a vehicle capable of making the trip to Denver.

I informed Jay that if he wanted to see our sons, he would have to agree to supervised visitation. He chose not to see them for the first couple of years. When he eventually resumed visits, I would drop the boys off at his brother's house so he could spend time with them there. Jay and his family had lived in Denver for several years while Jay was growing up, and his brother had returned to the city as an adult. He was a successful businessman with a great family, and I knew my sons would be safe at their house. Most importantly, I didn't have to have any direct contact with Jay.

I had lived paycheck to paycheck in Laramie, and now, with the cut in pay and the move to a much more expensive city, I teetered on the brink of financial disaster. Full-time child care for two children, an apartment, and other living expenses consumed most of my income. I begged Jay to send what little support he could. "Even five dollars a month will help buy milk," I pleaded. Jay still lived in Laramie and as far as I knew continued to work construction, but he refused to provide any assistance. I continued to live the spartan, desperate existence familiar to so many single moms.

Safehouse was located in a big, shabby old house on a busy street in the gritty Capitol Hill neighborhood just east of downtown Denver. The organization had gone through a period of serious mismanagement and had closed down temporarily, with the staff laid off, just before I was hired. I learned about the precarious financial situation only after I had been hired and moved my children to Denver. I still would have taken the job even if I had known earlier, because I really had no other options. After about three months on the job, I met with the board chair and several executive committee members. I told them I thought the organization could be brought back from the precipice, but it was going to be very tough, and a lot of people were going to be unhappy with me. I needed to know if the board would support my efforts. They gave me their word, and they upheld that promise through the ensuing months as I restructured the organization over the objections of the staff, while meeting with multiple funders. I assured our funding sources that we would be more accountable in the future and asked them to help us through the difficult days ahead.

Like many battered women's shelters, Safehouse opened in the late 1970s, as the civil rights movement made the natural progression to assisting women. In 1978 the US Commission on Civil Rights held its "A Consultation on Battered Women" hearing in Washington, DC. That effort eventually culminated in President Jimmy Carter's creation of the Interdepartmental Committee on Domestic Violence and the Office on Domestic Violence, which were comprised of representatives from twelve federal agencies. With recognition, cooperation, and advocacy at the federal level, battered women's shelters won some legitimacy. Funding, always a struggle, was vastly improved. However, with the election of Ronald Reagan as president in 1980, the Office on Domestic Violence was dismantled, and hard-won federal funds were discontinued.[1] Many start-up battered women's programs were shuttered, either temporarily or permanently.

Safehouse, like all battered women's shelters at the time — and most today — limped along for several years with too many clients and too little money. The board and staff were deeply divided. Leadership, often ineffective, changed frequently. I came in as an experienced and competent nonprofit manager, something Safehouse desperately needed, making me a godsend for the organization.

Safehouse was also a godsend for me. Despite the years of abuse, a stay in a shelter, and my struggle to free myself from Jay, I still didn't understand that my situation was mirrored over and over, in home after home, city after city. At Safehouse I began to see how closely my story tracked the stories of all the women who came through our shelter doors. At first, when I met the young women and their children living in the shelter, my reaction was that they should find good men to marry. I wondered how they could possibly make it on their own. Getting away from my abusive ex-husband was the most difficult thing I'd ever attempted; yet I had an education, a supportive family and friends, and job skills. These young women had several children each, little education, and no job skills. How could they possibly overcome such odds?

From these young women I learned that given time, a desire for change, opportunity, and options, people are able to overcome almost anything and even thrive. A loving husband or spouse is a wonderful thing, but not essential to a rich and fulfilling life. Each woman was eventually accepted at Warren Village, a transitional apartment community offering child care and case management. Warren Village gave these women the support they needed as their children grew a little older and they developed skills to support their families.

But these women were lucky; Safehouse counselors helped them to access the complex network of agencies and services necessary to help build new lives for themselves and their children. Every one of these programs operated with lengthy waiting lists, and all were extremely difficult to access. And services were available in Denver that often weren't available in other cities across the nation. Warren Village, in particular, was a unique program started by a local church. It had not been replicated elsewhere, and the services it provided were essential to achieving independence. I saw that it was possible for the overburdened system to work, but it was highly unlikely.

I remained close to several of these young women as they moved through Safehouse and into Warren Village. I visited them in their affordable apartment homes, conveniently located near downtown Denver. Licensed child care was available in the building, as were many other services, all of which, including rent and child care, were paid on a sliding-fee scale based on income. The women could live at Warren Village for eighteen months to two years while working to meet the objectives for independence they each established with their assigned case managers. I sometimes thought how much easier my life would be if I could live in Warren Village rather than my affordable but distant suburban apartment, where I drove my children daily to two different child-care programs. Those child-care programs consumed fully 60 percent of my income. If I lived at Warren Village, maybe I could afford to have my hair trimmed professionally or buy clothes someplace other than discount or secondhand stores. Yet each of these women was being given a hand up in hopes they could create a life like mine. And each of us readily affirmed that our lives were far better now than they had been when we were living with domestic terrorism, the threats and assaults of our ex-husbands.

Knowing these women helped me to know myself better. One, a red-haired, freckled earth mother, had been horribly abused her entire life. She married her abusive husband to escape her abusive father, a man who brought his drinking buddies home on Friday night and regularly offered up his twelve-year-old daughter as a sexual partner to them. We know this as gang rape, but the horror of a father as the instigator is almost unthinkable. I realized I was extraordinarily lucky to have a father who always adored, loved, and protected me.

Another was an elegant and self-assured black woman who saw abuse in her home growing up and came into the shelter pregnant with her third child. I realized I wasn't the only woman to be battered during pregnancy. In fact, it was a common experience. She wanted to have her tubes tied after the baby's birth; the public health-care system would pay for the birth, but not for elective sterilization. We raised the money to help her pay for the procedure.

Another woman was close to my age and reminded me of myself, a white woman from Middle America. She thought she came from a relatively normal family and was a smart, pretty, charming people-pleaser. She, like me, didn't understand how she had gotten into her situation.

I also remember Anne, a striking young woman whose father was the mayor of a suburban Denver city. She married her football-hero sweetheart from high school. Anne was white, he was African American, and her family disapproved. They had four great children, but the marriage was abusive. Because of her family's disapproval, this woman had no one to turn to when things got bad. She was a model shelter resident, doing everything possible to free herself and her children from her abusive husband. One summer afternoon, when she believed her husband was at work, Anne went home to pick up some belongings. Her husband showed up, held her hostage, and beat her until their children's pleas convinced him to let her go. She returned to the shelter, her clothes torn, her face bruised and bloodied. With her permission we promptly called the police. When the police came to take the report they first ran a check on her name and discovered that she had an outstanding traffic ticket. Given her circumstances, it was clearly impossible for Anne to have paid any fine, but instead of writing the report on her assault, the officers put her in handcuffs in front of her children and took her to jail for the unpaid ticket. And we questioned why women didn't call the police? In this instance, I was able to call a Safehouse board member, a captain in the Denver Police Department, to explain what had occurred. Anne was promptly released from custody, and the chief of police wrote her an official apology. He followed through on his promise to change procedures and provide training for officers responding to other such cases. Anne's ordeal served to help women who made the same call in later years.

I began to share my own experiences with the clients at Safehouse, but I continued to be cautious about opening up to the staff, primarily social workers. While professing to support an "empowerment" model of services, like so many professionals they tended to discount input from those who had lived the issue. Nor did I ever speak about my former life with the board of directors.

Together with the Safehouse board chair, Dave Weaver, I was helping to bring Safehouse back from the brink. Dave worked tirelessly as a volunteer to help rebuild the agency. Funding and staff were steadily increasing and improving, and previously suspended programs were now expanding and growing. Dave was the first of many special male volunteers I came to work with and count on in the years ahead. He was a single professional man, a successful entrepreneur who had no discernible reason to work for a battered women's shelter except for an enormous heart and the time and capacity to assist us. From the moment I took the job in Denver, he was one of the people I could count on. He was there to help unload my U-Haul when I first arrived from Laramie, and he continued to offer his thoughtful assistance when needed.

When I moved to Denver, my mother came to stay with me for several weeks so I could get organized and find care for my sons. She also provided a measure of comfort and a feeling of safety. At one point she took my sons and went home to Kansas for a few days, leaving me alone for the first time in years. The first night I came home from work to an empty apartment I feared that Jay might have tracked me down and was waiting for me inside. I sat in the parking lot for a long time, and I finally called a high school friend, former pro football player Bill Larson, who had lived in Denver for many years. I asked if he would come over and go inside with me to check the apartment before I stayed there alone. I knew I was being silly, but I couldn't shake my fear. Carrying a baseball bat, Bill checked every closet and under every bed. I was safe, but it would take me years to begin to accept and feel that safety as my reality. I later figured out that my illogical behavior was most likely associated with post-traumatic stress disorder. Research has shown that more than 60 percent of women who have sought refuge at battered women's shelters meet the criteria for post-traumatic stress disorder. Their hearts race. They relive the abuse in vivid dreams that rob them of sleep. They are always on guard, even when their abuser is nowhere near, even if he's in prison or jail. They don't have the comfort of escaping to their own homes to hide from their inner war zones.

As I began to see how my experiences mirrored the experiences of women entering Safehouse, I blamed myself less and felt more comfortable speaking out. When I quit blaming myself, I also quit expecting others to blame me. Many people still looked at me and at other victims and assessed blame. I no longer accepted that judgment. I finally started speaking out because it was clear to me that the general public believed domestic violence didn't happen to people like me. Men battered women who were poor, black or brown, uneducated, unassertive, and dependent. Blaming the victims is so much easier when those victims can be categorized as different or in some way less able than oneself.

I also began to discern the magnitude of the problem. Once I started working for Safehouse, people began sharing their stories with me unsolicited. The guy who came to install my phone told me about his concerns for his sister. The fellow across the hall cried as he described his mother's life. My dental assistant told me about her first marriage as she cleaned my teeth, and my son's teacher asked for advice about how to deal with her abusive boyfriend. These were the same kinds of people I had known and interacted with my entire life, but now that I worked at Safehouse they started talking to me about the domestic violence impacting their lives and the lives of their loved ones.

Looking back at incidents from my youth, I began to realize that unrelated events were part of a larger societal pattern. There was the neighbor in Wichita whom our family considered snooty; her home was always clean, her hair and makeup perfect, and she kept to herself. But her perfection crumbled the night she ran screaming and crying into the night in a torn nightgown, fresh bruises just beginning to emerge, begging the neighbors to let her into their house before her husband found her.

I remembered a grade-school friend who lived across the street and had, once again, the seemingly perfect family. They lived in a pristine, new, two-story house on a street of crumbling old bungalows. My friend talked in her sleep one night, in a tent full of friends on a Girl Scout camp out. She begged her father to leave her alone, to stop touching her, crying for her mother to please protect her from her father's advances. We listened, mesmerized, not realizing what we were hearing until many years later. Not one of us sought out a group leader, told our parents, or in any way responded to her plea for help.

I also recalled a girl in my seventh-grade English class who didn't come from the perfect family. She lived in a poor neighborhood, wore hand-me-down clothes, often missed school, and struggled to keep up with her classes. One day she told me that she and her sisters slept behind multiple locked doors in an effort to keep their father from attacking them in the night. Again, I never spoke up to tell anyone. I knew the father's behavior was wrong, but I didn't think I should become involved, and I didn't quite understand what she was trying to tell me.

As I listened to the new stories, remembered stories from my past, and began to understand the abuse in my own life, I realized it was past time to shine a light on the dirty little secret of the violence happening behind closed doors in supposedly idyllic homes. I first "came out" at an annual luncheon of the Mile High United Way, a major funder of Safehouse services. United Way representatives asked if I could find a battered woman willing to share her story at the luncheon, their biggest event, usually drawing up to a thousand participants. I said I could.

The courageous shelter client who spoke that day told of finding her former boyfriend hiding under her bed with a gun, intent on killing her when she fell asleep. But she was African-American, she had little education, and she was not married to her batterer. Although they recognized that she needed help, the affluent professional crowd in the room easily dismissed this woman as different from them.

In my introductory statements, however, I said I was a formerly battered woman who knew the courage it took for this woman to stand up in front of a crowd and tell her story. That was the extent of my remarks, but even as I said those two sentences I knew my life was again changing forever. I have been stepping forward ever since, but it has never been easy. I have braced myself at a podium in front of a thousand people while telling my story, all while my legs trembled uncontrollably. I have felt a whole new terror, the sense that the crowd felt nothing, as though the walls absorbed every emotion in the room except mine. As I have shared my story, I have again felt the shame, the hopelessness, and the fear that I would not be believed.

But people did believe me, and I slowly began to regain some measure of self-assurance. I also began to have a social life. I dated a police officer, perhaps recognizing unconsciously that a man who carried a gun for a living could protect me from Jay. We married after three years. For weeks before our wedding I suffered nightmares about Jay surprising me, stalking and hurting me. The day after we married, to the astonishment of both of us, I recoiled with physical fear when my new husband turned suddenly to speak to me. He never once threatened me or raised a hand to me, but despite years of safety fear still shadowed my life.

We stayed married for almost a decade. We moved to Texas together, first to Fort Worth and then to Austin, his hometown. Together we had a beautiful daughter, Megan. He was often away from home because of his job, and I had a demanding and high-profile job that consumed much of my time and energy. Our interests diverged. This book isn't about that marriage, but I recognize now that the marriage was based more on my history, weaknesses, and fears than on the person I was becoming. The more I healed and embraced my strengths and accomplishments, the less the marriage seemed to work. I am the one who changed, but I would never go back to being the frightened, insecure woman I was when we first met and married.

In July 1993 I took over as executive director of the Center for Battered Women in Austin. This time, I stated up front that I was a formerly battered woman. I said I would bring my experiences as a one-time shelter resident and a survivor to the job of running the organization, and if that wasn't okay with them, then I wasn't the right person for the job. I guess the board recognized that my personal experience, coupled with my nonprofit-management experience, could be an asset, because I was hired.

Arriving in Austin to run the Center for Battered Women was totally different from my arrival in Denver. I was now secure in my ability to run the agency. I knew I could make it in the big city, and I didn't feel I needed to hide a part of my past. Even then, the Center for Battered Women was a nationally recognized program with a strong board and staff and secure funding. I knew I had just grabbed the brass ring of jobs in battered-women's programs.

3

defining
the problem
of domestic abuse

A spaniel, a woman, and a walnut tree,
the more they're beaten, the better they be.

— Old English proverb

I REALIZE NOW HOW LUCKY I WAS TO ESCAPE FROM LARAMIE with my life. Jay's behavior mirrored warning signs of a harasser bent on deadly violence; studies of women killed by intimate partners identify common traits among perpetrators, and Jay was classic. He had access to a gun, he had already threatened me with a weapon, we were estranged, and he stalked me. He battered me when I was pregnant with our child. He also abused drugs and alcohol, and he was chronically unemployed.[1]

Every day, domestic violence takes the lives of four women in this country. In the dry language of social scientists, a woman is far more likely to be killed by an "intimate acquaintance" or another family member than by a stranger. That means husbands, common-law spouses, and boyfriends are murdering women at an appalling rate. Almost one-third of female homicide victims reported in police records are killed by an intimate partner.[2] According to the Violence Policy Center's (VPC) report on a full range of gun violence issues in the United States, in 2004 more than nine times as many women were killed by guns clutched in the hands of men they knew than were killed by unknown men. Male acquaintances of women claimed 1,587 victims. We warn our daughters to lock their doors and watch out for strangers, but VPC statistics show that male strangers killed only 168 women that year.[3] We should be educating our daughters about how to detect red flags signaling potential violence in the men they already know.

I repeat, I was lucky to get away from Jay with my life. I also was lucky that the abuse was bad enough for me to recognize that my life and health would be in danger if I were to stay and continue to "try to make the marriage work." Before my marriage to Jay, my father had no conscious understanding of battering. As I revealed the horror of my marriage, however, he began to see how abuse had impacted the relationships of other women he loved. He once described another relative as a battered woman. "He controls her with money, doling it out bit by bit, never providing enough to cover even the bare necessities," he said. "He belittles and berates her; he attacks her self-esteem, calling her fat, ugly, worthless, and worse. He humiliates and insults her in front of family and friends, keeps her from working, and threatens to take custody of the kids if she ever tries to leave him. But she will probably stay forever, because he doesn't hit her or hurt her physically." My father was right: She was indeed a battered woman and she would stay in the marriage, never being forced to acknowledge the constant barrage of verbal and emotional assaults she endured on a daily basis.

In my years of working with victims of domestic violence, I have found that almost universally an abused woman will tell you that the battering of her self-esteem is far more devastating than the physical abuse. The assaults are more insidious, subtler, and more difficult to assess and escape. Whereas some emotionally abusive relationships don't involve physical abuse, all physically abusive relationships contain some emotional abuse. And although bruises heal, the assaults on self-esteem may last a lifetime.

It has taken me more than two decades to talk about the emotional and verbal abuse that obliterated my self-esteem when I was married to Jay. Even now, as a happily married woman and an accomplished professional, I feel humiliation and fear that someone reading this will look at me as damaged goods. When I was a young mom going through a divorce, Jay's verbal assaults caused me to isolate myself, building a wall of fear between myself and other men. Besides constantly telling me I was unattractive, Jay ferociously attacked my sexuality. Cody's birth was difficult, resulting in a rectal–vaginal fistula, a tear between the rectum and the vagina. This sort of injury occurs mostly in impoverished Third World countries, usually in very young women whose bodies are not ready for childbearing. The condition was embarrassing beyond words and not something I could talk about with others. Surgery repaired the tear, but Jay insisted I was permanently damaged. He referred to me as "canyon cunt," and said I could never please a man because "your hole is like a giant cavern." I now know that a loving and respectful partner in a healthy relationship would never say such things. These verbal attacks were more powerful and effective in Jay's efforts to control me than any physical assault I endured.

But how does battering in a relationship or marriage differ from the marital spats and disagreements that almost all couples engage in?

Understanding the answer to this question is key, because not all men who occasionally lash out at their wives should be defined as batterers. We will never win the battle against domestic violence until more people understand that domestic abuse is *abuse,* plain and simple.

In broad terms, battering is the use of force or coercion by one partner to maintain power and control over the other partner. "Power" and "control" are the key words, because abusive relationships are never based on mutual respect. The use of force or coercion can include not only physical assaults, but also verbal, sexual, economic, and emotional abuse. And it is important to understand that battering is a pattern of behavior, not an isolated incident. One partner repeatedly asserts control and ownership over the other, through whatever means necessary. By convincing me I was undesirable to other men, Jay got his way. He kept his stranglehold on me, even when we were no longer married. Although I fled the marriage, he achieved his goal. He made sure I stayed away from other men.

Sadly, most people do not have a clear understanding of what constitutes abuse. They believe someone must be bruised and bloodied to be a victim. There have to be multiple calls to the police, as well as visits to the emergency room. A doctor's X rays should document the abuse, showing a cracked jawbone or a broken arm. A black eye is almost mandatory. But it isn't always necessary to use physical violence to establish ownership and maintain control over a partner. Just the threat of violence, or of losing economic support or one's children, is often sufficient to keep a partner in a constant state of fear and subjugation. Unfortunately, this kind of abuse — the malignant shadow of violence — can be difficult for a woman to articulate. When she dreams of escaping, she is reluctant to turn to a shelter, reluctant to take a bed from a woman who is "really" abused. Like all battered women, she thinks she won't be believed — and she doesn't have the X rays, the black eye, or the police reports to support her case.

Historical Perspective

Some men believe they are supposed to control their wives. In their minds, the end justifies the means. Often, they have learned violence in their families, and sometimes in their societies. Religious beliefs may convince them they must control their wives; perhaps they embrace St. Paul's admonishment that wives should submit to their husbands while ignoring Jesus' commandment to "do unto others as you would have them do unto you."

Violence against women and children has continued through the millennia because of beliefs that give one person or group of people power and control over another person or group of people, and these beliefs need to be confronted. Abuse of women is historically echoed in abuse of blacks, abuse of Native Americans, and abuse of workers. A culture that systematically denies the value and rights of ethnic minorities, the elderly, the disabled, gays and lesbians, women, and girls creates a society that spawns abuse of women and children.

Sometimes, men don't want to hear about the issue of domestic violence because they think all men are being attacked. That isn't true; history records many stories of respectful and fair treatment of women, even in societies saturated with the belief that women should subjugate themselves to men. Still, for whatever combination of reasons, some men turn violent, and at least in our society these men are different from the norm. They abuse the power that history and culture have bestowed upon them. That's why all men need to learn about the violence that can harm their own mothers, daughters, and sisters, and why we need to examine the history of the subjugation of women.

Patriarchal cultures have provided the seedbed from which domestic violence has grown, and the three great bodies of thought that have influenced Western society's views and treatment of women all assume patriarchy as natural. Greek philosophy, Judeo-Christian religious ideas, and the common law legal code all promoted male domination of women because males were viewed as superior.[4]

"Greece of the eighth through the fifth century BCE was a thoroughly patriarchal society. Women's legal and social subordination was undisputed," reports Dr. K. J. Wilson in her book *When Violence Begins at Home*.[5] In Will Durant's *The Greatest Minds and Ideas of All Time*, the Greek philosophers Plato and Aristotle both make his top-ten list of the people who have most influenced worldview[6] — and both defined women as "inferior" creatures in need of being controlled. Aristotle expressed the generally held view of women when he wrote, "The male is by nature superior, and the female inferior; and the one rules, and the other is ruled; this principle, of necessity, extends to all mankind...the courage of a man is shown in commanding, of a woman in obeying."[7] Plato wrote, "Of those who were born as men, all that were cowardly and spent their life in wrongdoing were transformed at the second birth into women.... Such is the origin of women and all that is female." However, Plato also wrote, "If women are expected to do the same things as men, we must teach them the same things," making him very progressive toward women in his day.[8] These ideas were carried into Roman culture; husbands were legally entitled to chastise, divorce, or kill their wives for engaging in behaviors such as drinking from the family wine cellar or walking outdoors with their faces uncovered.[9]

In some Jewish and Christian interpretations of the Old Testament, women were associated with serpents and sin, viewed as innately evil. Eve lured Adam to eat the forbidden fruit, causing the fall of man and "original sin." For centuries, the stain of original sin was used as justification to subjugate women to the authority of the church, state, and men, and much of early common law was based upon the church's teaching. God's punishment of Eve required that she obey her husband, codified by the law's sanction that husbands rule their households and impose "moderate" correction.

The common law system, established in England in the eleventh and twelfth centuries, set the precedent for American, Canadian, and Australian rules of conduct governing marriage for many centuries to come. Wives were viewed as their husband's property, and laws governed men's control of that property, ensuring wives' obedience. But these laws weren't limited to countries deriving their law from the English system. In sixteenth-century Russia, the murder of one's wife was legal if committed for disciplinary purposes. The Russian Orthodox Church gave its blessing to the law with the publication of the "Household Ordinance," an edict outlining how best to beat one's wife.[10]

The subject of women's inferiority and their need to be obedient dominates many pamphlets and manuals written during the middle of the last millennium. The sixteenth-century Protestant reformer and scholar William Tyndale, in *Obedience of a Christian Man*, instructs husbands that "God which created woman, knoweth what is in that weak vessel and hath therefore put her under the obedience of her husband to rule her lusts and wanton appetite."[11] Legal guidelines were developed allowing a husband's instrument of correction to be as thick as a man's thumb, purported by some to be the origin of the phrase "rule of thumb."[12]

One form of domestic abuse, marital rape, was considered an oxymoron — and still is considered so by some. Marital rape in the United States was first outlawed in 1978 in New York State when a statute was passed that prohibited forced sexual intercourse by a stranger, an acquaintance, or a spouse.[13] By 1993, all fifty states had laws on the book against marital rape. However, thirty-three of the fifty states continue to regard spousal rape as a lesser crime than nonspousal rape.

Susan Brownmiller, in her book *Against Our Will: Men, Women, and Rape*, reports, "Female fear of an open season of rape, and not a natural inclination toward monogamy, motherhood or love, was probably the single causative factor in the original subjugation of woman by man, the most important key to her historic dependence, her domestication by protective mating."[14] But in her pursuit of protection from rape, a woman paid a high price; she gave over ownership of her body, offspring, and property to her so-called protector. Thus, the rape of women was long considered an offense primarily against men, who were deemed to be the wronged parties. Rape was only secondarily judged an offense against the woman who was raped. Punishment and compensation for rape depended on the degree to which the crime affected the interests of the father or the husband of the victim and damaged the value of the man's property (his wife or daughter). The original US rape laws, some of which weren't changed until the 1970s, defined the crime of rape and its penalties in terms of the "crime" against the husband or father of the victim. In many jurisdictions, rape laws were similar to those regulating cattle theft. The legal system did not conceive of rape as a crime against the woman herself. This state of affairs continues to exist in countries and cultures that condone so-called honor killings.

The tendency to devalue women and view them as property has led to a variety of unspeakably cruel practices, including foot binding, witch burning, chastity belts, clitoridectomies, and infibulations. In much of the world—and in our own history—violence against women has actually been encoded into a society's rules of conduct. Foot binding in China ensured female chastity by, among other things, ensuring that women literally could not "run around."[15] Thankfully, this custom is only a bad memory. Often, however, a ritual is so deeply ingrained in a culture that it is difficult to erase. This is the case with the Hindu practice of "sati," or widow burning. Written accounts exist describing the horror of sati in northern India as early as the fourth century BCE.[16] As recently as the early nineteenth century, the province of Bengal officially recorded the occurrence of 7,941 sati rites, of women throwing themselves, or being thrown, onto their husbands' funeral pyres to be burned alive.[17] The practice was outlawed in British India in 1829 but continued well into the twentieth century until the Rajasthan Sati Prevention Act of 1987, which made abetting a sati, directly or indirectly, subject to a death sentence or life imprisonment.[18]

Whereas foot binding and sati have been abolished, many cultures, groups, and religions continue to enshrine systems and beliefs damaging to women and girls. One of the disastrous unforeseen impacts of the war in Iraq has been a rise in the number of honor killings, which have reportedly increased by the hundreds since the 2003 invasion. Yanar Mohammed, 2004 president of the Organization of Women's Freedom in Iraq, reported that ten years ago honor killings had been completely eradicated in Iraq. By 2008 authorities in the southern Iraqi city of Basra admitted they were powerless to prevent these so-called "honor killings," following a 70 percent increase in religious murders during the previous year.[19] In 2007 the *National Catholic Reporter* described how a seventeen-year-old Iraqi girl was stoned to death by the men of her village for the offense of fraternizing with a boy from another religion. As she was tortured, male onlookers cheered and took pictures with their mobile phones. The police stood by while other men raped the girl for the sake — they said — of restoring their own honor.[20] Baby girls are still murdered in parts of China and India simply because of their gender, and female genital mutilation continues to be practiced by some African, Indonesian, and Middle-Eastern cultures.[21] This barbaric custom involves the surgical removal of the clitoris and the closure of the labia majora by sewing them together to seal off the genitalia, leaving only a small opening for the passage of urine and menstrual blood. The Office of the United Nations High Commissioner of Human Rights estimates that around 130 million girls and women worldwide are currently subjected to this torture.[22]

All around the world, women and girls are raped, battered, tortured, and killed. The World Bank estimates that violence against women is currently as serious a cause of death and incapacity among women of reproductive age as cancer, and is a greater cause of ill health than traffic accidents and malaria put together. Besides being a fundamental violation of human rights, violence against women represents one of our most critical public health challenges and is a major factor contributing to poverty.[23]

Despite the fact that the United States is considered a developed nation and a world power, only in the last half century or so have laws and customs begun to recognize women as valued individuals, instead of mere property. This change is due in large part to the feminist movement that first emerged in the late 1800s and then re-emerged in the 1960s and 1970s. I have lived in a time in which I have been able to observe a monumental shift in women's rights in America. I am fifty-four years old as I write this. My mother is seventy-four, and my daughter is nineteen. My mother came of age in a time when women weren't allowed to hold credit in their own names, there was no effective method of birth control, and abortion was illegal. I have watched as the women of my mother's generation fought for the rights and freedoms that my daughter and her friends enjoy, even take for granted, and I have seen some women grow old and embittered by their lack of opportunity.

These are the women who opened doors for my daughter. The girls of her generation have grown up with few memories of the severe restrictions and limitations my mother's generation fought to overcome. They believe they can hold any job open to their male counterparts. An African American woman has held the position of Secretary of State, and a woman much like their mothers holds the highest office in the United States House of Representatives. In one generation the US population has evolved from one in which women were far less educated and represented in the work force than men, to one in which half the work force and more than half of the college population is female.

I grew up knowing women who had fought hard for the right to vote, a right young women take so much for granted today that they often forsake their duty to influence the democratic process. My grandmother White, a schoolteacher and a widow from a young age who raised two of her three children mostly as a single mother, told how her uncle, Albert Houston Roberts, a former governor of Tennessee, risked his political life to ensure that women, including his sister — my great-grandmother — would have the right to vote. That was less than a century ago. Women activists endured beatings, public humiliation, and forced feedings as they worked to mobilize the country behind the nineteenth amendment. Although many men fought against women's suffrage, it was also men, since they were the only ones with the power to vote or hold office, who eventually stepped forward on their side. My great uncle Albert was one of them.

Albert Houston Roberts took office as the governor of Tennessee in 1919, the year Congress passed the nineteenth amendment. It needed to be ratified by thirty-six states. By August of 1920, thirty-five states had signed. If not ratified by one more state before the end of the year, the amendment would die. Sentiment ran against the amendment in the remaining states, mostly in the South and the West, and no state legislature was scheduled for session before the end of the year. According to family lore, my great-uncle passionately believed that women should vote. Many in the Tennessee legislature, however, thought giving women the right to vote would result in moral decay and the end of the United States as a great country. They believed that women were to be controlled and obedient. Furthermore, Roberts was embroiled in a tough re-election campaign, and his advisers warned against his calling a special session over such a divisive issue. But Roberts called the session anyway. And then he traveled the state, pulling in favors and using every bit of his influence to force the issue. History was made when the measure passed the Tennessee legislature by one vote.

Tennessee's capital, Nashville, crawled with reporters, and all eyes were focused on the state. The White House and the Tennessee governor's office exchanged telegrams daily. On 24 August 1920 my uncle signed the bill. Two days later, women earned the constitutional right to vote. Roberts isn't mentioned in any history books, he failed in his bid for re-election, and he never ran for office again. When he was considered for inclusion in Kennedy's *Profiles in Courage*, he missed the cut. But my grandmother, Mildred Justice White, credited her mother's brother when she first stepped into a voting booth.

I have been accused of being a "crusader," a designation used as an attack, but one that I accept with pride. My great-uncle Albert was a crusader who stood for what he believed in and did the right thing. We have come far in our work toward acknowledging, valuing, protecting, and honoring the contributions of women and girls. But our work isn't nearly done.

The Victims

Battering is largely a crime of violence perpetrated by men against women. The US Department of Justice reports that women make up 84 percent of spouse abuse victims and 86 percent of victims of abuse at the hands of a boyfriend or girlfriend. Women between the ages of twenty and twenty-four are at the greatest risk of experiencing nonfatal intimate-partner violence.[24] The United Nations Population Fund reports, "This gender difference appears to be rooted in the way boys and men are socialized — biological factors do not seem to account for the dramatic differences in behavior in this regard between men and women." Let me repeat that: *Biological factors do not seem to account for the dramatic differences in behavior.* That's important because given the awful history and prevalence of violence against women, one might be tempted to think violence is inevitable, as natural as the sea pounding on the shore.

Nearly one in four women in the United States reports experiencing violence by a current or former spouse or boyfriend at some point in her life.[25] The Department of Justice reported in 2005 that women are much more likely than men to be victimized by a current or former intimate partner. Women make up 84 percent of victims of spousal abuse and 86 percent of victims of abuse at the hands of a boyfriend or girlfriend, and about three-fourths of the perpetrators of family violence are male.[26] In addition, male violence against women does much more damage than female violence against men, for obvious reasons: Women are much more likely to be injured than men because men are typically bigger and stronger.[27]

Still, men can be and sometimes are the primary victims of domestic violence. After all, abuse of power is the real issue. In the National Violence Against Women Survey, approximately 23 percent of men reported being raped, physically assaulted, and/or stalked by a male intimate partner. Seven percent of men reported such violence by a wife or female cohabitant.[28] Men, however, are more likely to be financially independent and therefore less likely to fear leaving a violent relationship. They are also less likely to seek emergency shelter or other such services.[29] Unfortunately, when men do find themselves the victims of domestic violence and need protective shelter, they often have no place to turn. They may be unable to access the shelter network. Many shelters do not provide services for men, and those that do seldom publicize that fact adequately.

At SafePlace, in Austin, we became painfully aware of our oversight when a young man, Albert Woods, was tracked down, shot, and killed by a male partner he was attempting to leave. The responding officers found a SafePlace brochure on his kitchen table. We wondered why he didn't avail himself of our services. We learned that Albert had talked with the police department and a volunteer from victim services, but no one referred him to our shelter. When we asked why he was not referred to the shelter, the response was, "Because you don't take men." At that time we operated out of a building with shared bedrooms and communal bathrooms, so it wasn't possible for us to shelter men there. We did, however, work with hotels to place battered men in vacant rooms. At the same time that Albert was murdered by his former partner, we were sheltering another man with his children in a local hotel.

This tragic occurrence caused us to take a critical look at our printed materials and the way we discussed our services. We realized we consistently referred to our program as a "battered-women's" shelter and spoke of men as perpetrators and women as victims. Furthermore, until we merged with the Austin Rape Crisis Center in 1998, our organization was called the Center for Battered Women. We immediately corrected our printed materials to ensure gender neutrality where possible and to state clearly that our services were also available for men who were victims of battering. When we were able to design and build a new shelter facility, we incorporated a small efficiency apartment for use by battered men and other clients who might need special accommodations.

Underreporting of Violence Against Women

As I've pointed out, batterers almost always count on their partners' silence. Jay didn't deny the violence when I told my story to the judge; he merely expressed amazement that I'd spoken out. Battering has historically been considered "a family matter," and research continues to indicate that the crimes of domestic violence and sexual assault are dramatically underreported.

The National Institute of Justice found that 73 percent of domestic-violence incidents go unreported. I would assert that the incidence is even higher. Sexual assault is reported even less often. Every year some 132,000 women report to law enforcement that they have been victims of rape, but in a national victimization survey administered by the Bureau of Justice Statistics to approximately 77,200 households in the United States on the frequency of crime victimization, as well as characteristics and consequences of victimization, 42 percent of respondents said they told *no one* about the assault. Only 5 percent reported the rape to the police.[30]

Indicators of an Abusive Relationship

The first step toward reducing domestic violence is awareness and recognition of the warning signs of an abusive relationship. A potentially abusive partner may embarrass his partner by using bad names and putdowns; look at her or act in ways that scare her; control what she does, whom she sees, whom she talks to, or where she goes; and stop her from seeing or talking to friends or family. An abusive partner may take his partner's money, make her ask for money, or refuse to give her money. He may make all the household decisions and prevent her from working or attending school. He may tell her she's a bad parent or threaten to take away or hurt their children. He may act like the abuse is no big deal or is her fault. He might even deny doing what he does. He may destroy her property or threaten to kill her pets. He might intimidate her with guns, knives, or other weapons. He may shove her, slap her, choke her, or hit her. He may force her to have sex. If she files charges, he may force her to drop them. He may threaten to commit suicide, or to kill her.[31]

Every one of the behaviors listed above is a red flag for a potentially abusive relationship. However, most battering doesn't begin with forced sex, choking, or threats of suicide or death. Most battering begins with more subtle controlling behaviors: excessive jealousy, isolation from other friends and family, belittling and bullying, or destruction of property. If most battering began with black eyes and broken bones, fewer women would stay in the relationships past the first incident. But because battering most often starts with jealousy, and many girls and women confuse jealousy with love, they stay, believing, as I did, that intense jealousy signifies intense love.

Many women have also learned through their cultures or families that abuse in a marriage is the norm. In April 2008 Texas Child Protective Services took more than 460 children from the Yearning for Zion Ranch, in Eldorado, Texas, into state custody. I volunteered to provide assistance. The Yearning for Zion Ranch is a compound built to house members of a breakaway Mormon sect, the Fundamentalist Church of Latter Day Saints (FLDS). Members of the FLDS believe in plural marriage, and there is considerable evidence that underage girls at the ranch were being forced to marry much-older men. I was asked to host one of the young mothers in my home.

(My offer met with very mixed reactions from my children. My son Cody, now a young man, asked why I would agree to such a request. "Why don't you just take in a battered woman, or something like that?" he asked. I said, "This is the ultimate battered woman, someone who has never even had the opportunity to learn what she can be.")

A young woman whom I will call Abby came to stay with me. She was both everything I expected and nothing at all like what I expected. She would have adamantly denied that she was a battered woman in any way. She would have said that it was her choice to be a part of the FLDS church, to live at the ranch, to be the third or fourth wife of a much older man, and to live under the rigid rules dictated by her "omniscient" husband and the prophet. She was a terrified, naïve young woman who had little experience with the outside world. She had been raised in Hilldale, Utah, as a member of a multigenerational FLDS family. At one point, Abby asked me what I thought of them and of her. I told her that my goal was to provide her with a safe and comfortable place to stay while she worked toward getting her children returned — that it wasn't my place to judge her. However, I said, the children at the Yearning for Zion Ranch lived such an insular life that they didn't have the opportunity to make a choice about the church.

Despite her protestations, I believe that Abby never had a choice either. She had learned the lesson through her church and her family that women and girls were possessions to be controlled. Still, Abby put her role as a mother first. She said that if she were forced to choose between her church and her children, she would absolutely choose her children.

Battering and Child Abuse

Like most battered women, I left my marriage many times before I was finally able to break away for good. And like many mothers, I finally took the steps to leave for good once it was clear to me that my children were being hurt by the violence. Many people express surprise when they hear that SafePlace, like almost all battered-women's shelters, actually shelters more children than adults. The majority of women seeking shelter come with young children. And almost 100 percent of the time those children have also experienced abuse, either as spectators or as victims.

The US Advisory Board on Child Abuse suggests that domestic violence in the home may be the single major precursor to child abuse fatalities.[32] According to the Judicial Council of California's Center for Families, Children, and Courts, child exposure to domestic violence is estimated to have a 40 percent co-occurrence with some form of child maltreatment. Other research has found the overlap between child abuse and domestic violence to range between 30 and 60 percent. In addition, in a national survey of more than six thousand American families, 50 percent of the men who frequently assaulted their wives also frequently abused their children.[33] Child abuse is almost universally recognized as a crime, and wife abuse should be viewed with equal abhorrence.

Women who are battered will often go to extreme lengths to protect their children from an abusive partner. Research has shown that the nonabusing parent is often the strongest protective factor in the lives of children who are exposed to domestic violence. SafePlace has historically sheltered a greater number of abused children than any other program in Central Texas, including the Children's Shelter. The primary difference is that abused children being sheltered at SafePlace have the benefit of at least one parent who is trying to protect them.

Even for children who are not being physically abused, growing up in a violent home may be a terrifying and traumatic experience, affecting every aspect of a child's life and growth. Infants exposed to violence may fail to develop the attachments to caretakers that are critical to their development; in extreme cases they may suffer from "failure to thrive." Preschool children in violent homes may regress developmentally and suffer sleep disturbances, including nightmares. School-age children who witness violence exhibit a range of problem behaviors, including depression, anxiety, and violence toward peers. Adolescents who have grown up in violent homes are at risk for re-creating the abusive relationships they have seen.[34]

Luckily, children are resilient, as evidenced by the success of my own sons and the many stories of the children who came to SafePlace. We knew we were achieving some success in our programs for children the night a neat, well-mannered, articulate young man in our volunteer-training program introduced himself to the rest of the group and explained his personal reason for engaging as a volunteer. "As a kid, I lived for two months in that corner bedroom with my mom, brother, and sister," he said. "This place saved my life, and now I want to give something back."

Battering and Alcohol and/or Drug Use

An enduring myth, one that is exceedingly difficult to dispel and one that I myself once believed, is that alcohol and drug abuse *cause* battering. I wanted to believe that Jay wouldn't hit me if I could just keep him from drinking. But even after he quit drinking, his obsession with me, as well as the stalking and battering, continued. I sat with him in an Alcoholics Anonymous meeting as he stood up and announced to the group, "I am an alcoholic and I abuse my wife." The group applauded his ability to recognize and name his behavior, while neglecting the reality that just describing himself as a batterer wasn't sufficient to address and change that behavior. We now know that being drunk or high is most often an *excuse* for abusive behavior, not its cause.

However, while substance abuse is not generally the primary cause of domestic violence, there is a statistical correlation between the two.[35] Studies of domestic violence frequently indicate high rates of use of alcohol and other drugs by perpetrators during abuse.[36] Moreover, a battering incident that is coupled with alcohol abuse may be more severe and result in greater injury. The US Department of Justice found that 61 percent of domestic-violence offenders also have substance-abuse problems.[37] Furthermore, adults with childhood abuse histories have been found to have more severe substance abuse disorders, to have started using at a younger age, and to use substances for reasons that differ from other clients.[38]

Substance abuse can exacerbate violence against women and children, and vice versa. They should be treated simultaneously, but they rarely are.[39] The failure to deal with domestic violence in substance-abuse programs or to deal with substance abuse in domestic-violence programs interferes with the effectiveness of both programs. Many service providers recognize the correlation between the two issues, but few domestic-violence programs can offer adequate counseling or health services for substance abusers. "Limited resources" is the main reason cited for the absence of substance-abuse-treatment programs in connection with domestic-violence programs, because resources are necessarily focused on providing safety and shelter. However, 80 percent of programs that cannot provide substance-abuse-treatment programs for victims or abusers do refer these people to substance-abuse-treatment programs in their communities.[40]

Jay's treatment for substance abuse was successful as far as it went. To my knowledge, he quit drinking and stayed sober. And even though the abuse didn't stop, I personally benefited greatly from my involvement with Jay's treatment. At some point in the process I picked up the Al-Anon book *One Day at a Time in Al-Anon*. I read that book every day for a long time, asking God to "grant me the serenity to accept the things I cannot change, the courage to change the things I can, and the wisdom to know the difference." I had spent years believing I could bring rationality and sense to a crazy situation, that I could in some way make things right or make Jay understand how irrational he was being. I credit the principles of Al-Anon with helping me to see I had no control over his actions and could not change them or him.

While I applaud the tenets and successes of Alcoholics Anonymous, Narcotics Anonymous, and other twelve-step programs, I continue to encourage them to expand their horizons and recognize that addiction and violence are not synonymous. While one may be held in abeyance, the other can still rear its ugly head unless there is specific intervention to address both issues. My good friend, Mack Martinez, Travis County Attorney in charge of domestic-violence prosecutions and protective orders, talks of repeatedly seeing NA and AA compatriots step forward to provide testimony and alibis for friends who were eventually found guilty of serious domestic-violence and protective-order offenses. Later, the friends report having been duped, saying, "I knew he was staying clean, so I didn't think he could have done the other."

The Intersection Between Domestic Violence and Sexual Assault

Domestic violence also correlates strongly with sexual abuse and assault, because both are essentially issues of power, control, and dominance. Both are also crimes primarily committed by men against women and children. In America, one in six women and one in thirty-three men have experienced an attempted or completed rape.[41] The US Department of Justice has estimated that fifteen percent of victims of sexual assault are under age twelve and 44 percent of rapes occur before the victim is age eighteen.[42] Ninety-three percent of juvenile sexual assault victims know their attacker.[43]

When Safehouse in Denver first hired me, the staff told me that as many as 50 percent of the clients they served had been sexually abused as children. As with so many things, I immediately discounted their statements — I thought it just wasn't possible. I later came to understand that battered women who were molested as children are often in the most dangerous relationships, with no family support system they can turn to for help. Fifty percent of battered women are not survivors of childhood sexual abuse, but these are the women most often seen in shelters because they must rely on community and governmental support systems for assistance, and those systems often fail.

Those of us who work to end rape, sexual abuse, and domestic violence have long recognized that childhood sexual abuse is often at the root of many of society's most intractable problems. Alcoholism, drug abuse, eating disorders, homelessness, and welfare dependency have all been linked to childhood sexual abuse. What's more, a 2002 report by the World Health Organization reported that victims of sexual assault are three times more likely to suffer from depression, four times more likely to be suicidal, and twenty-six times more likely to abuse drugs.[44]

A report titled "Sexual Assault in America," published in 1995 by the American Medical Association, uncovered disturbing attitudes among youth toward sexual violence. In a survey of high-school students, 56 percent of the girls and 76 percent of the boys believed that forced sex was acceptable in some circumstances. A survey of male college students found that 35 percent anonymously admitted that they would commit rape under certain circumstances — in other words, if they believed they could get away with it. One in twelve admitted to committing an act that actually met the legal definitions of rape, and yet 84 percent of men who committed rape did not label the act as such.

Even more disturbing were the attitudes of youths aged eleven to fourteen, gleaned from the same study. Fifty-one percent of the boys and 41 percent of the girls said forced sex was acceptable if the boy "spent a lot of money" on the girl. Thirty-one percent of the boys and 32 percent of the girls said it was acceptable for a man to rape a woman with past sexual experience. And 87 percent of boys and 79 percent of girls said sexual assault was acceptable if the man and the woman were married.[45] This survey is now fifteen years old. My most fervent hope is that we have made headway in changing some of the attitudes it reveals.

I believe one of the strengths of SafePlace is its mission to end both sexual and domestic violence, a mission arrived at through a merger of the Austin Rape Crisis Center and the Austin Center for Battered Women. The combining of these two programs, finalized in 1998, was twenty years in the making. Both agencies dealt with problems of violence against women and children that were primarily rooted in issues of power and control. Both worked closely with the criminal-justice system and other victim service agencies. Both educated health-care providers to improve their awareness of and response to victims of violence. Both worked with schools to develop and provide violence-prevention programs for youth, both operated twenty-four-hour crisis hotlines, and both provided extensive group and individual counseling programs. So why did it take so long to merge the two?

The staff and volunteers of the Austin Rape Crisis Center were concerned that the issue of domestic violence would overshadow the issue of sexual violence. I admit to being arrogant and thinking, "They just don't know how to talk about it in a way that people can hear what is being said. They are too strident and accusing. I can do this so that people will hear."

I was wrong. As the executive director of the merged agency, I found that the media, politicians, and the community in general prefer to deny the pervasiveness and destructiveness of rape and sexual abuse. No matter how hard we try to highlight the issue of sexual assault, to this day SafePlace is typically described as a "battered-women's shelter." We very purposely changed all of our language to highlight the rape and sexual assault components of SafePlace services. Despite this disparity and our efforts to address it, bringing the issue of sexual assault to the forefront continues to be a struggle. And incest and child sexual abuse continue to be almost invisible.

This very invisibility is what allows abuse to flourish and spread like a virus, infecting children, families, and communities. Violence begets violence, creating patterns that multiply across generations. As I learned and spoke about the prevalence of family violence, my own relatives began to talk about domestic abuse in our family history, events that for years had remained secret. The depth of the infection became apparent.

generations

In the beginning, when my mother started speaking out, I was embarrassed. I didn't want anyone to know that stuff. I thought it was personal and I didn't know why she should be sharing it with anybody, especially strangers.

— Daughter of a domestic-violence survivor

ONCE I STARTED TO BREAK THE SILENCE SURROUNDING THE abuse in my marriage, I learned that my experience was not an anomaly. Stories of physical and sexual abuse that permeated generations of my mother's family began to leak out. It is difficult to fully know a story that spans a century or more and is shrouded in family secrets, and it is almost impossible to determine what is real and what is imagined. I have heard it said that "our sickness is in our secrets," which explains a lot about the persistence of domestic violence through generations of families. Understanding how a disease spreads is an essential component of its treatment and eradication, and domestic violence is one of our society's most pervasive and insidious behavioral diseases.

Tracing the Roots of Violence in My Family

My maternal grandmother, the woman I considered a second mother for most of my childhood, told me that her first husband, Larry, came home from days away spent driving a truck and regularly turned his rage against her. She told me that the day she made him leave for good, she had a black eye and a swollen face from the previous night's beating. She also told me that Larry had a "girlfriend at the other end of the line."

I have been told that Grandpa went to California and never returned to live in Kansas. He essentially disappeared from my mother's life. He married again — more than once — and fathered additional children, half-siblings to my mother. No one in my family has ever met them. Through the grapevine, we learned that one of his wives packed up everything and left while he was at work. While in the Navy, my brother met someone who might have been his half-uncle, but the man refused to speak to him. For the next fifty years, my mother diligently checked the white pages in every town she visited to see if her father's name was listed.

My mother loved her father and never understood why he left her to be raised alone by her young, lonely mother, a woman who supported herself and her daughter as a grocery store clerk. Her memories of their time together as a nuclear family are bleak. My mother told me that when she was four or five years old they lived in an aged motel room while my grandmother worked at a chicken farm plucking feathers. Grandpa was unemployed.

I met my maternal grandfather only once, when I was five years old, and I have no more than vague memories of his visit. I remember my mother's lighthearted anticipation and a rare happiness suffusing our home while he was there. A photo from that day, of my beautiful young mother with her five small children and her handsome, tall, dark-haired, bespectacled father sits on my mantel. My sister remembers that he bought presents for each of us — she got a doll's highchair, and my mother got the fancy high-heeled shoes my father couldn't afford. After a short visit Grandpa left, never to return again. When he died, an old and broken man living alone in a trailer in California, he left a small inheritance for my mother. It turns out that he had established a trust fund into which he put most of his retirement pay, ultimately amounting to a tidy sum. I have often thought how much more her father's presence in her life would have meant to my mother than the money he left her.

Mother resented my grandmother for the breakup of the marriage and for her manic hunt to find another man to take my grandfather's place. The hunt was not necessitated by economic need; my grandmother always worked and provided adequate support for herself and her daughter. The desperate search came from my grandmother's need for a man in her life to make her feel whole. Night after night, my mother was left alone as my grandmother, made up and dressed in gaudy and provocative clothing, set out for an evening of dancing and drinking. My mother speaks bitterly of the humiliation she felt as her mother caroused in search of a man to take my grandfather's place. My grandmother was a divorced woman at a time when divorce was rare and shameful, and most other moms were home preparing meals, keeping the house clean, and helping with their children's homework; thus, my mother's mother was living a life that was quite scandalous for the time.

My grandmother eventually remarried and had another child, my uncle Pat, only six months older than I and younger than my older sister. Our family practically lived at their house for much of my youth, and my uncle was more like a sibling to us. My grandmother settled into domesticity, but she didn't spoil her grandchildren because she was a mother herself and still working. By that time she was a steady, reassuring presence in our lives.

My grandmother's second husband, Vincent, was a veteran of the bloody Pacific beaches of World War II. He soothed his torturous memories with drink, eventually losing his job because of alcoholism. My most vivid memories of Vincent are of a quiet, even morose, man who sat endlessly in his recliner in front of the television, a cigarette in one hand and a can of Coors beer in the other. Sometimes he let me taste the beer. I also remember him occasionally catching me in his legs in "a bear trap," the most animation I ever saw from him.

His drinking was yet another family secret I didn't understand until I was an adult trying to make sense of how I could have been so blind to Jay's substance abuse. As a child I never wondered why Vincent didn't go to work during the day like other men. When I was a thirty-something single mother, my mother and grandmother finally told me about finding bottles of vodka hidden in the basement rafters after Vincent's death from lung cancer.

In fact, my extended family was remarkably adept at keeping secrets. Those secrets, many only addressed years after the fact and others never discussed to this day, clearly crept into my subconscious and informed my strategies for living. From past masters, I learned to keep secrets and protect those I loved from public scrutiny.

My grandmother also began to talk to me about her own mother and father. Everyone had always told me I reminded them of my great-grandmother Annie Duckworth Woods, a tall, raw-boned woman who bore twelve children, nine daughters and three sons. Two of the sons died while still young, but all nine daughters lived long lives. Some of my great-grandmother's children were younger than my mother. Grandmother Woods was born in the Missouri Ozarks, a once-remote region settled by pioneers from Appalachia. These were people accustomed to hardship, who figured a difficult life was their due and asked for no more. According to a family history written by my great-grandmother's sister, the children walked to church barefoot, donning their shoes when they reached the outskirts of the church clearing. My great-great-grandfather kept his savings under the porch steps, but he donated land to build the local school.

My great-grandmother's height — she was six feet tall — was apparently viewed as an impediment to her finding a husband. When a stranger came to her tiny hometown flashing a roll of twenty-dollar bills, the family was encouraged that he showed interest in "Amazon Annie." They urged her to marry the short, skinny stranger, John Woods. Annie wed the flashy outsider, and they moved west to homestead in the Colorado sand hills. You can't farm sand, so they continued their journey. Because they were desperately poor, they traveled in a covered wagon when others were crossing the prairie by car and train. They eventually settled in western Kansas, where the family lived hand-to-mouth while my great-grandfather worked as a farmhand and my great-grandmother took in laundry and ironing.

My great-grandfather has been described as "a mean little man" who brutally beat his wife and all of his children. I never heard a single one of his children say a kind word about him. When speaking of him, all of them used words like "evil," "violent," and "mean." My grandmother rarely spoke about her father. Once, she said he suffered from "terrible headaches," although he had "a singing voice like an angel." John Woods' nine daughters held him in particular contempt. My grandmother told me he repeatedly molested his "favorite" daughters. My grandmother, always a tough, smart survivor, said she escaped the worst of his abuse because he didn't perceive her to be as pretty or malleable as some of her sisters. Life at home was so bad that every daughter escaped as soon as they were able, marrying young and starting families of their own.

Most of the nine sisters are now dead, and I only have remnants of memories of my grandmother's stories. She told me about Lucy, our favorite great-aunt, who married her husband after knowing him only a week. Together they reared four children. We all adored her husband, a charming and funny man, who swept her off her feet in a romantic, fairytale love story. What we didn't know was that he drank too much and that he physically and verbally abused her and their children. As an adult running a battered-women's shelter, I was amazed to open a popular women's magazine and see a story written by my great-aunt Lucy's daughter. She detailed her struggles as a battered woman and the eventual suicide of her ex-husband when she refused to return to him. In his suicide note he blamed her, saying he was killing himself to get back at her for leaving him.

Jenny Sue, another great-aunt, was always considered the most beautiful of the daughters. Unfortunately for her, her father also noticed her beauty, and my grandmother said he particularly doted on her. She was the recipient of his unwanted and devastating sexual advances. Jenny Sue left home as soon as possible, marrying a man she later divorced while he was in prison. Even a priest had insisted she must divorce the man, who was violent and abusive. Jenny Sue went on to have, by all accounts, a successful second marriage.

The details of my mother's father's life are even murkier. He was one of eight children, five brothers and three sisters, who grew up on a farm in northeastern Kansas. My grandfather and many of his brothers were very handsome. Although I have never seen her picture, his mother was said to be an exquisitely beautiful woman. Over my years of working with battered women I have come to view beauty combined with lack of power as a curse. What I have put together from bits and pieces of information is that a streak of instability ran through my maternal grandfather's family. My father described "Big Ed," my mother's grandfather, as mean and given to violent mood swings and erratic behavior. I don't know for sure that he was violent; no one else has told me that, because the few family members I knew would never talk about him. My great-grandmother, however, divorced him sometime before 1930, despite having eight children.

Almost by accident, I learned that one of the eight children, a great-uncle from my maternal grandfather's family, ended up sending his child away to be raised elsewhere after his wife was killed in a mysterious "accident." Just a few years ago my sister was surfing a genealogy website when she ran across a thread clearly pertaining to my mother's family. Someone was searching for foster children placed with a St. Louis family many, many years ago. The foster children would have been my mother's cousins. Somehow, one cousin found the missing foster children, and a reunion came about. One of them, a cousin named Judy, told a strange tale. "I was just three or four years old," she said. "My mother died, and I started telling people, 'Daddy hit Mommy with a beer bottle, and she didn't get up,' and I was immediately shuffled into foster care."

⌒⌒

My father's family was very different. His mother was a schoolteacher and his father always worked steadily, even in the 1930s when people were leaving the Great Plains in droves because of the Dust Bowl and the Great Depression. My grandfather White, legendary for his industriousness, retained his job as district manager for a farm equipment manufacturer at the same time that almost everyone else — including his salesmen — joined the ranks of the unemployed. My father said that during the worst of it he remembers his father being the only one of his friends' parents who had a job.

World War II interrupted their seemingly idyllic life. My father's older brother, my uncle Joe, joined the military and was shipped overseas. Daddy, approaching adolescence, stayed at home with his mother, father, and younger sister, Nancy. Not long after the war ended my grandfather went into the hospital for some minor surgery. During the operation he suffered a heart attack and died at the age of forty-three, leaving my grandmother to raise my father and aunt Nancy alone. She had no insurance and had not worked in years. She never remarried, once saying "she couldn't imagine crawling into bed with another man."

Mother and Daddy began dating in high school and spent the rest of their lives together. Unfortunately, Daddy's upright family disapproved of his relationship with the girl from, quite literally, "the wrong side of the tracks." The family that valued education and financial and professional stability didn't give her a chance, and I think my grandmother White blamed my mother for my father's choices, considering it my mother's fault that he married right out of high school, forsook the chance for a college degree, and devoted his life to trying to support his five children.

These choices also engendered significant conflict between my parents. I have memories from my childhood of my father coming home late after a night of drinking and of my mother's fury. I remember nights huddled in fear under the bedcovers as vicious battles raged in the room down the hall. As a child I never saw much evidence of love between my mother and father, but I learned well the lesson of perseverance, of playing the hand you're dealt. And I am grateful my parents chose to play the hand they were dealt. They were barely able to support their five children, and I don't doubt we would have spiraled into even worse poverty had they split up in those early years.

In addition to the volatility and strain in their marriage, their struggles to make ends meet, and the animosity between my father's family and my mother, their first son was critically ill from the day he was born. My brother Steve was born just one year and two weeks after me, and he suffered from a mysterious malady that affected his ability to digest and absorb food, necessitating multiple long stays in the hospital as an infant. He was diagnosed with cystic fibrosis, and my parents were told that he wouldn't live past his early years. Needless to say, my parents had no health insurance, and things seemed to be about as bad as they could get.

Much has been written about the dynamics of a family with a critically ill child, and my family was true to form. Most of my mother's time was spent dealing with Steve's doctor appointments, hospital stays, special dietary needs, and medications. She was always exhausted and afraid of what the future held, and the birth of my twin brothers when Steve was a year and a half old didn't help. In a home with too little money and attention to go around, those resources became even scarcer.

The conventional wisdom is that siblings of children with chronic or serious illnesses can be "forgotten" while the family is focused on the sick child. That can cause resentment, anger, anxiety, depression, jealousy, fear, and guilt in the children who are lucky enough to enjoy good health. These days there is a lot of awareness among professionals about the impact of a sick child on siblings, and hospitals even offer programs for the healthy kids. We, however, grew up in the days before "psychology" was daily television fare. Children like us often felt isolated, unimportant, and afraid of upsetting our parents even more. And children with a sick brother or sister sometimes see the benefit of having their own problem of one kind or another. I learned that the best way to get the notice of my harried parents was to have something go wrong. In a family that reeled from crisis to crisis, I unconsciously incorporated the notion that living in catastrophe was the norm. I think we all did.

Having a sick sibling can also have some positive effects, and again we were true to form. Siblings of a child with a chronic illness tend to be more compassionate, understanding, and sensitive. Often they are more resilient than other children. Other troubles seem trivial.

Steve defied the doctors' predictions and lived to adulthood, dying from AIDS at age forty-one. My parents, however, reared him with the certainty that he would be dead within the next few years. So while my brother lived, he was raised as a dying child, which helped to define both the dynamics in my family and my personal strategies for managing my life.

As I've said, my father never hit my mother or any of his children in anger. In general, he was kind and gentle, especially with us kids. Yet I believe that I was in part socialized, by my early years as the sibling of a chronically ill child and by the history of my extended family, to be open to the attentions of an abusive man and to accept his abuse as my fault. I had also become accustomed to living on the edge — teetering near the precipice, becoming addicted to the adrenaline surge, trying to avert the next crisis. Somehow, in my world it wasn't okay for me to be successful and happy and to dream about — let alone hope to achieve — the prosperity and accomplishments I want for my children.

More important, and harder to explain, was my transformation from a victim into an empowered woman who looks to her own inner resources for happiness and fulfillment. I walked away from my identity as someone who waited for a knight in shining armor to rescue her and make her life better. I am no longer that woman.

I grew up watching *Queen for a Day*, one of the most popular television shows of the 1950s and 1960s. One of the original reality-TV shows, it featured four contestants competing to be crowned Queen for a Day based upon their personal tales of woe, which were disclosed to a live audience of hundreds and an electronic audience of millions. Using a classic "applause meter," the studio audience voted for the contestant who came closest to hitting rock bottom. *Queen for a Day* turned the tradition of Horatio Alger on its head. Instead of a boy or girl making good, the woman who told the story of the greatest hardship—the tear-jerk factor was critical—would be crowned to the accompaniment of "Pomp and Circumstance." The winner was draped in a red velvet robe, and a shimmering crown was placed on her head. She received trips, a fully paid night on the town with her husband or escort, and other prizes. Critics accused the show of exploiting the women who competed, a charge I think bears up. But even worse was the model it set for girls: the worse your life, the better your chance of being rescued. Fairy tales and other children's stories of the era conveyed the same story: A damsel in distress rescued by some beneficent force beyond herself—most preferably a handsome man.

Don't get me wrong; I don't think I was led to an abusive marriage because of a television show or my family's difficulties or any one experience I can point to. Still, I do believe that each of us is primarily a sum of our parts—the experiences and factors that have molded who we are and how we live our lives. And I believe that we are molded by attitudes and beliefs passed down through generations, not just behaviors.

As I have tried to understand my own part in an abusive marriage, I have sometimes been accused of "victim blaming," of taking partial responsibility for what someone else did to me. This is not so. Blaming the victim releases the man who commits violence from the responsibility for what he has done. But if we hope to end violence against women, it is essential that we change not only the behaviors of the perpetrators, but also the behaviors that have sometimes made the victims vulnerable to an abusive relationship.

My most important healing occurred years after my final break from Jay, and I don't think it would have happened had I not serendipitously

stumbled into the battered-women's movement and eventually internalized the lessons for living an empowered life. My life and future changed
at the point when I quit thinking of myself as a victim and stopped looking to the crises and problems in my life to define me—the point at which
I quit daydreaming about being crowned Queen for a Day or being rescued by a knight in shining armor. True empowerment is the goal for
all formerly battered women and the programs that serve them, but it is
often elusive, both individually and organizationally.

Generational Patterns of Abuse

Studies show that witnessing violence between one's parents or caretakers is the strongest risk factor for transmitting violent behavior from one
generation to the next.[1] Violence begets violence. Men who witnessed
domestic violence as children are twice as likely to abuse their own partners and children as are the sons of nonviolent parents.[2] And women
who were abused as children are more likely to become victims of abuse
as adults.[3]

An oft-told SafePlace success story perfectly portrays these genera-
tional patterns. One morning, SafePlace staff who worked with violence
prevention in elementary schools received a frantic phone call from a
school social worker. Five first-grade boys had just chased down a first-
grade girl on the playground, pulled down her pants, and tried to sexually assault her. SafePlace staff arrived to find all five boys and the girl
gathered together in the principal's office for a "problem-solving" session. Our staff immediately pointed out that the girl was not a part of the
problem; just like a young woman blamed for being raped because she
was wearing a short skirt, this little girl had not brought the assault on
herself. In addition, arrangements were underway to transfer the little
girl out of the classroom—yet more evidence that she was being identified as *the* problem. Luckily, as soon as these things were pointed out,
everyone recognized the flaws in their logic and quit treating the girl as a
part of the problem.

Of equal concern to the SafePlace staff were the little boys who had
engaged in such an aberrant activity, particularly the boy who was identi-

fied as the ringleader. Where could he have learned this behavior at such a young age? The staff met with the parents as they came to pick up their children, including the mother of the leader. When she heard what had occurred she sobbed that it was her fault; her son was only doing what he had seen at home. He was doing exactly the same thing that he saw his father do to his mother. This little boy was lucky. His mom immediately left her husband, came into the shelter with her son, and received counseling for years. I have lost track of the child, but I can only hope that he learned a different way to be in the world.

Some of the finest men I have ever worked with in my efforts to end violence against women grew up in violent homes. They talk of finally being able to stand up to their fathers in defense of their mothers. And they are exemplary husbands and fathers. Prisons are full of men who were abused as children, but not all men who were abused as children grow up to be violent. Nor do all women who were victims or who witnessed abuse as children grow up to be abused. There are no set rules for human behavior. We want answers and neat categories, but all we have to work with are imprecise patterns, suggestive trends, and possibilities.

Internalizing Empowerment, Both Individually and Organizationally

Battered women, and the women and men who have dedicated their lives to helping them escape from violence, are some of the smartest, toughest, and most resilient people I have ever met. But many have been socialized, like me, to expect the worse and to think that living from crisis to crisis is the norm. This has often been evident in management of the organizations developed to address the issue. One of the main reasons for the success of SafePlace has been its ability to transcend victimization and work to incorporate the concept of empowerment into the organization's structure.

Shelter for battered women has been provided, since the earliest times, by women, often women who recognize the need because they have seen and experienced abuse themselves. These are women who have usually been told they "aren't good enough" and have lived with crisis for so long that it has become their norm. This crisis condition is often incorporated into the running of the programs. Every battered-women's program has operated from inception with too little money, too many clients, too much drama, and too little security. The challenge of these agencies is to transcend the "victim" mentality and operationalize empowerment, just as this is the challenge for the women who come through the doors.

How, you ask, can this be accomplished when, in fact, you *are* operating a crisis program and there *is* too little money and there *are* too many clients, many dealing with life-and-death issues? The reasons for operating in crisis are all very real. I eventually learned that one of my most important tasks as a manager was to be a leader; my job was to model consistency and stability and to de-escalate crisis situations. I learned to surround myself with the very best people, people smarter than me; to listen to their thoughts, ideas, and concerns; and to manage for the best among us rather than the worst among us. We trained and recognized people for using good judgment, we learned from our mistakes, and we moved on. People devote their time and energy to working in programs dedicated to ending domestic violence and sexual assault because they want to create a better, safer world. People will work for money — but they will give their lives for meaning.

5

who is
at risk?

Battering happens everywhere,
anywhere, not just to women in
poor neighborhoods. It happens
in nice neighborhoods. It happens
in families that look like happy
families—like mine.

—A survivor

WHEN I WAS WORKING IN DENVER I MET A YOUNG WOMAN who used a wheelchair because her legs were paralyzed from an accident in her youth. She was working hard to organize a victim-support program for people with disabilities, a project she initiated after a stranger broke into her home and raped her. As a relative newcomer to the world of victim's services, I remember being completely flabbergasted and horrified to learn that a perpetrator could commit violence against someone so obviously defenseless. I have since learned that, yes, predators do walk among us. They seek as their prey those perceived as weak and vulnerable, just as the big cats of the African veldt search for the young or the injured to cut from the herd and attack.

The Austin SafePlace shelter housed a young woman with developmental disabilities because members of her family—her primary caregivers, charged with loving and protecting her—were physically attacking her. The woman, in her mid-twenties but functioning more like a ten- or eleven-year-old, also suffered from a serious seizure disorder that sometimes required hospitalization. One night, uncontrolled seizures precipitated her transportation by ambulance from the shelter to the hospital, and her case manager hurried from home to meet the woman there. Before the case manager arrived, but after her seizures had abated, the young woman was left alone in the emergency room waiting area. While she waited, and unbeknownst to anyone, a lurking predator recognized her vulnerability and lured her from the crowded emergency room to a secluded area nearby, where he sexually assaulted her.

After her assailant fled, the woman wandered back into the waiting room, dazed and disheveled. When her case manager arrived at the hospital, the woman told her what had occurred, a story reinforced by her appearance. She couldn't provide many specific details, and her assailant was never caught. Since that incident, the SafePlace shelter, which struggles to provide adequate staff coverage for the overnight shift, always asks clients needing to go to the emergency room via ambulance (whether they have disabilities or not) if they would like to be accompanied. If the person wants company, sometimes a staff member accompanies them. Sometimes another client goes along.

Although anyone can be battered, some people or groups of people seem to be more vulnerable to victimization than others. Society, ethnicity, family, or other circumstances mold the predator/prey relationship.

I was a white, well-educated, middle-class mom, and yet I was a victim of domestic violence. There is no point in overrationalizing the reasons why someone becomes a victim, because not everyone fits into a tidy mold. Nevertheless, we must do more to ensure that people whom we know are at high risk have access to needed resources and services when they are hurt by violence. As a society, we also need to hold perpetrators accountable for their actions.

Studies have confirmed that if you are poor, black, or brown, you are more likely to become a victim of intimate-partner violence. You are at increased risk if you are pregnant or have a disability. Researchers have also found that victims often are troubled by poor self-esteem, depend on the abuser for economic and emotional support, and nurture unrealistic beliefs that the abuser will change. They believe that jealousy is proof of love.

Violence Against People with Physical and Developmental Disabilities

Wendie Abramson, director of disability and deaf services at Austin's SafePlace, says that when she was deciding to take the job, a supposedly knowledgeable person asked, "Who would want to hurt someone in a wheelchair?" Wendie says the remark has stayed with her through her years of working to end violence against people with disabilities. She had been employed by the local United Cerebral Palsy agency and has dealt with the conundrum faced by adults with disabilities who are abused by their caregivers. Should they live with fear and abuse, or give up the dependable care that often has made it possible for them to live independently and hold a job? In every case, victims said they wanted to maintain the caregiver relationship. They just wanted the abuse to stop.

Few people want to admit that violence against people with disabilities exists, but denial of the problem has allowed the abuse to fester. Many police departments, shelters, and other social-service agencies are simply unprepared to deal with violence against people with disabilities. I remember with regret deciding against repairing an elevator in a Denver shelter I managed in the mid-1980s. We were short on money — as always — but the elevator provided the only way for a person with a physical disability to reach the shelter facility, which was located on the second and third floors. My justification: "No one using a wheelchair ever comes into our shelter, and I need to use that money elsewhere." Clearly, no one using a wheelchair ever came into our shelter because they quite literally could not get into the building. My ignorance and arrogance got in the way of my good sense.

Violence against people with disabilities is almost always about asserting and maintaining power. Whatever the relationship between perpetrator and victim, it bears all the hallmarks of intimate-partner violence. The abuse is used as a means of demeaning and controlling the person with disabilities.

Very limited research exists on the extent of violence against people with disabilities, and many studies are outdated, but available research and anecdotal observations support the claim that people with disabilities are more vulnerable to being victimized. When victimized, some are unable to advocate for themselves because they are often totally reliant upon their perpetrator for food, personal care, health-care support, and other vital services. They may lack access to a telephone or a way to independently get out of the house.

In addition to physical, verbal, and sexual abuse, perpetrators may abuse people with disabilities by overdosing or withholding medication, stealing money, denying necessary equipment, and forcing them to remain immobile. The disability may even be a result of prior abuse. Denver's Domestic Violence Initiative found that 40 percent of women with disabilities who sought the agency's services had acquired a disability as a direct result of domestic violence.[1] Independent of age, race, ethnicity, social class, or sexual orientation, women with disabilities are raped, assaulted, and abused at double the rate of women without disabilities.[2]

"Crimes and violence against people with disabilities are an invisible epidemic," writes Daniel D. Sorensen, former chair of the California Coalition on Crime Against People with Disabilities. According to Soren-son, these crimes include rape, assault, and murder, as well as economic crimes. "Most experts agree that the rate of violent crime is from 4 to 10 times higher for people with disabilities than for the general popu-lation," he writes. "An estimated 31 percent of all personal crime com-mitted in California is committed against people with substantial dis-abilities. Studies have found that from 83 percent to 90 percent of women and 32 percent of men with intellectual disabilities have been sexually assaulted. However, this disproportionate concentration of violence is largely invisible to our society, partly because these crimes are severely under-reported. Fewer than 5 percent of personal crimes against people with disabilities are reported in California, compared to over 42 percent of such crimes against people without such disabilities."[3]

I began my career working with people with disabilities, and yet I was completely ignorant about the abuse they so often endured. When I was a young occupational therapy intern at a rehabilitation hospital in Chicago, a patient told me that her husband said she shouldn't come home since she was now "only half a woman." A middle-aged wife and mom, she had undergone a hemipelvectomy—removal of her entire pel-vis and one leg—in an effort to arrest the spread of a particularly virulent type of cancer. Her prognosis for long-term survival was grim. I now think that the husband's words and actions were a particularly hideous type of abuse, attacking both her self-esteem and her sexuality. In an in-cident revealing a somewhat similar mindset, a friend lost her lower leg in an automobile accident when she was just out of her teens. She is now an accomplished adult, but she is still haunted by the fact that her parents sued the other driver, in part because of their daughter's "loss of mar-riageability."

I have come to realize that, despite being professionally trained to work with people with disabilities, I understood little about the culture and sensibilities of the disabilities community. I have made mistakes throughout my career, some of them appalling. I continue to try to im-prove my sensitivity about these issues. To cite one important example, I have learned that words are important. Language holds tremendous meaning because it shapes attitudes. Advocates for people with disabilities have educated us in the social services to use "people first" language—that is, to emphasize the *person* rather than the *disability*. We are encouraged to say "person with a disability" rather than "disabled person" because most people with disabilities want to be thought of as ordinary individuals, defined by characteristics other than a disability. I have learned to try to emphasize abilities, for example, "uses a wheelchair" instead of "confined to a wheelchair" or "wheelchair bound."

At a SafePlace staff meeting several years ago I referred to "handicapped parking spots," not realizing that I was using terminology some would find demeaning. Within the day I was visited by a contingent of staff to educate me about the term "handicap" and why it is considered disparaging. Many disability-rights advocates hate the term "handicap." Some say it derives from the phrase "cap in hand," which refers to begging in the street—the only means of survival for people with disabilities in centuries past and, increasingly, today. I have read conflicting accounts of the etymology, but I no longer use the term because it is considered disrespectful and degrading to a significant number of people with disabilities.

I have found that if I don't know the right words or the correct actions, it is best to ask someone who does know. Sometimes I simply ask the individual I am dealing with. I have asked a person with blindness or low vision if they would like for me to assist them across the street. Once, I was in a conference with a deaf person who was assisted by a sign language interpreter, and I finally realized I should ask the deaf woman whether I should look at her or at the interpreter when I spoke. She said I should look her in the eye and speak directly to her, rather than to the interpreter, just as I would when meeting with anyone else.

When I speak about an individual who is deaf, I just say "deaf." That is the language the deaf community uses. The deaf and hard-of-hearing create their own communities, and most do not consider deafness a disability. They have their own language, culture, schools, and universities. While many deaf individuals prefer to work, socialize, and be educated among their peers who are also deaf, others choose to associate with and be assimilated into the "hearing" community. This can depend on whether they grew up in a deaf family, attended a school for the deaf, use sign language as their primary means of communication, and many other factors.

I have had ample opportunity to interact with members of the deaf community. Austin is home to the Texas School for the Deaf, a sprawling campus located just off of trendy South Congress Boulevard. More than ten thousand students have attended the school since its inception in 1857, and many have chosen to stay and make Austin their home, creating a large deaf and hard-of-hearing population and, ironically, creating challenges for domestic-violence and sexual-assault programs.

Austin's SafePlace has made determined efforts over the years to work with the deaf community by hiring deaf staff, providing free American Sign Language training for all SafePlace staff, providing signing interpreters for deaf shelter residents, and generally trying to work with the deaf community in whatever way is needed. Initially, SafePlace worked closely with an organization called DAWCAS (Deaf and Abused Women and Children's Advocacy Services) and incubated the agency by providing space in its facilities and administrative and program assistance. When DAWCAS was dissolved, SafePlace assimilated the majority of the specialized services for the deaf community into its portfolio of programs.

One of the challenges of working with the deaf community, and all communities made up of people with disabilities, is dealing with the close-knit nature of the group and the isolation associated with being a member of such a group. For one thing, the chance of maintaining confidentiality is limited. When working with the deaf community in Austin, we had to be careful when contracting with signing interpreters. We might utilize an interpreter with a relationship to one of the people with whom we were working, possibly violating confidentiality and putting the individual in further danger.

Some particularly egregious stories of violence against people with disabilities have gained national notoriety over the last few years, increasing the general population's awareness of the issue. The public was outraged by the gang rape several years ago of a young girl with a developmental disability by high-school sports stars, and more recently by the "fight clubs" organized by eleven employees at a facility in Texas, who forced residents with profound disabilities into late-night fighting bouts. But more of these cases go undetected than are spotlighted in the media. And even when the media momentarily shine a light on a particular incident, the common feature of violence perpetrated against people with disabilities is rarely identified and recognized as a plague further imperiling and destabilizing their lives.

Violence Against Women During Pregnancy

Women who are pregnant or newly parenting are particularly vulnerable to abuse. As a young pregnant woman I was appalled that my husband would abuse me. I thought this was a time when I would be cherished and adored, not hit and kicked. And I was certain that I was alone; surely no other husband and future father would treat his wife and unborn baby in such a brutal manner. Much later, I learned that pregnant and recently pregnant women are more likely to be victims of homicide than to die of any other cause,[4] usually at the hands of the men who professed to love them. During pregnancy, women are routinely screened for gestational diabetes, neural tube deficiencies, preeclampsia, smoking, and alcohol use. Research indicates that domestic violence occurs at least as often — if not more frequently — than these risk factors, yet health professionals are not screening for it.

Every year, between two and eight women give birth while living at the SafePlace emergency shelter, not an unusual rate for a shelter facility of its size. At any given time, 10 percent of shelter residents are pregnant and 10 percent of children living at the shelter are infants under the age of one. These women have all confirmed what research shows: Pregnancy is a time when risk of violence increases for women who are already experiencing domestic abuse. Those of us working in the battered-women's field know that there are two periods when battered women are in the most danger: when they leave the abusive relationship and when they are pregnant.

The danger also extends to the time following birth, when the batterer feels he is losing control over his partner. Her time and attention are no longer totally focused on him but rather on attending to the needs of the infant. One new mom came into our program after her husband had broken both of her thumbs. He told her, "See if you can change those diapers now!"

One morning I walked the hallways and rooms of the SafePlace shelter with Diane McDaniel Rhodes, then the director of residential services, trying to figure out what colors we should paint the walls. I noted another woman pacing the halls. I couldn't miss her because she was the most badly beaten woman I have ever seen. She wore a sleeveless shirt and shorts, and she was bruised on every visible part of her body. I was so disturbed by the degree of her injuries that I kept asking Diane, "Are you sure she's okay?"

"Yes," Diane reassured me. "She is okay, we are watching her."

"But why doesn't she lie down or something? She must be in pain."

Diane told me that the woman was walking at the recommendation of the hospital to try to induce labor. Black-and-blue from head to foot, she was also nine months pregnant, a fact that had totally escaped my notice because of the level of injury to her body, perpetrated by the father of her baby.

Violence Against People with Mental Illness

Doing this type of work, I think I have mostly learned to just expect the unexpected. One afternoon, two Secret Service agents arrived at the SafePlace administrative offices to investigate terroristic threats being made against the president of the United States by one of our residents. Another time, we received a phone call from a former client telling us she was in a van in our parking lot and was going to set herself on fire in protest of our denying her re-admission to the shelter. Both were individuals who, in addition to dealing with issues of abuse, were also dealing with severe mental illness, a regular occurrence within the world of domestic-violence programs.

Mental illness, as a type of disability, is often one of the most difficult issues for battered-women's programs to address, and the relationship between domestic violence and mental illness is extremely complex. Mental illness in either the victim or the perpetrator can be a risk factor for abuse, and mental illness in victims can also be an outcome of abuse. A significant number of people viewed as having a mental illness report histories of sexual assault, domestic violence, or other trauma.

In fact, experiences of abuse and violence are especially high for women diagnosed with serious mental illness. Numerous studies have indicated that between 40 and 70 percent of female psychiatric patients have been physically and/or sexually abused.[5] And, of course, some victims of abuse have been treated as mentally ill simply because they've come forward about the abuse. They have been locked up in institutions, their children have been taken away from them, they have been diagnosed with psychiatric illness, and they have been labeled for life. Once they're labeled, the focus shifts from the trauma to the psychiatric diagnosis.

Unfortunately, the typical social-service agency doesn't effectively screen for the intersecting issues of trauma and mental health, resulting in trauma survivors being moved from one mental-health facility to another, without ever addressing the underlying issues disrupting their lives. In a multisite study where 98 percent of people with severe mental illness (such as schizophrenia or bipolar disorder) reported at least one traumatic event, the rate of post-traumatic stress disorder (PTSD) was 43 percent. Nevertheless, only 2 percent of the people with PTSD had this diagnosis reported in their medical charts,[6] meaning other caregivers would be operating in the dark.

The mental and emotional distress faced by women experiencing serious abuse is overwhelming. In a study correlating domestic violence and welfare reform, almost half the women reporting serious domestic violence also met the criteria for major depression. One-fourth of them met the criteria for post-traumatic stress disorder.[7]

Battered-women's shelters are often as guilty as other social-service providers in failing to respond to abuse victims who deal with the two-headed monster of mental illness and domestic violence. However, as community mental-health services shrink and fewer insurance companies cover mental health, shelters must — by default — be able to respond more effectively to the requests for services from people who are doubly cursed.

One of the most pernicious aspects of the shrinkage in public and private dollars to fund mental-health services has been the corruption of the diagnostic systems. As the executive director of SafePlace I knew people whose diagnoses once qualified them for extensive medical and psychiatric services at the community level, ensuring them access to psychotropic medications and assistance to live independently in the community. Suddenly, their diagnosis was changed, and the powers-that-be deemed them well enough to live without the supportive services that guaranteed their independent survival. No, they were not miraculously cured. It was simply an underhanded way of moving them off the public-funded rolls. Denied the support that helped them to live independently, they often ended up moving back in with abusive family members or spiraling deeper into mental illness, ending up homeless on the streets.

In 2003 the SafePlace Disabilities Services Program conducted a national survey of domestic-violence and sexual-assault programs. Some 66 percent of respondents reported they served survivors with mental illness, compared to just 6 percent serving people with physical disabilities, 7 percent with cognitive disabilities, and 1 percent with sensory disabilities.[8] Responding programs also complained about their problems in adequately serving this population, prompting SafePlace Disabilities Services personnel to publish a manual, *Beyond Labels: Working with Abuse Survivors with Mental Illness Symptoms or Substance Abuse Issues.* It provides domestic-violence and rape-crisis-center staff with tools for working with survivors whose mental health has been affected by violence and trauma and who have coped with the violence by abusing drugs or alcohol. I recommend the manual to anyone dealing with these issues. It can be purchased through the SafePlace website, www .safeplace.org (see Resources).

Battering in the Lesbian/Gay/Bisexual/
Transgendered (LGBT) Communities

My brother Steve, born exactly one year and two weeks after me, was gay. His sexual orientation was the great "unspoken" in my family for many years. I think we all knew it, but we never talked about it. As a gay man, he experienced all of the ups and downs and trials and tribulations of anyone else in an intimate relationship. He moved to Florida as a young adult and became involved with a man I never met but with whom I think he was deeply in love. I also believe this lover was abusive. After a couple of years, Steve returned home to live with my parents, still denying his sexual orientation to his family and friends in conservative western Kansas. He was disconsolate, destitute, and suffering from a serious back injury. His lover called incessantly, twelve to fifteen times a day, and Steve slipped further into depression. We were all concerned for his mental and physical health.

After Steve had been home for several months, Daddy called me to tell me he thought Steve was suffering from a broken heart but didn't know how to talk to anyone in his family. My quiet, reticent father told me he thought the man who had been calling Steve was his former lover. This was the first time we ever spoke of what we all knew to be true. But none of us recognized he might have been fleeing an abusive relationship. Many years later, his new partner, Jonathon, told me about the abuse in the previous relationship. Once again, I hadn't been able to recognize abuse, even though it was an issue I dealt with daily in my work and had lived through myself. I think I was blinded by my own biases and expectations. But the LGBT communities have also hid the issue, primarily, I believe, because of a fear of homophobia and victim blaming.

"There are a growing number of studies providing estimates of the prevalence of violence within LGBT relationships, but results are currently quite limited," report Denise A. Hines and Kathleen Malley-Morrison in their book *Family Violence in the United States*. "The National Violence Against Women Survey (NVAW) contained an item where respondents indicated whether they had ever lived with a same-sex partner as part of a couple. Rates of intimate-partner violence were then compared between respondents with a history of same-sex cohabitation and those reporting only opposite-sex cohabitation. These comparisons revealed significantly more intimate-partner violence in the same-sex cohabitants than in the opposite-sex cohabitants. However, the abused women in same-sex intimate relationships were not typically being abused by their same-sex partners. Rather, intimate-partner violence against both male and female partners was most commonly perpetrated by men"[9]

Addressing domestic violence that occurs in lesbian relationships meets with some distinct barriers. Besides dealing with potential misogyny, the battered lesbian must face abuse within the context of a homophobic world. Even in the relatively informed environment of battered-women's shelters, battered lesbians can be met with disbelief. Women aren't supposed to be violent toward one another. Violence within the LGBT communities is further complicated by the response of law enforcement, prosecutors, judges, and service providers. Same-sex battering is viewed as "mutual battering" — another example of victim blaming and minimizing.

Victims within the LGBT community also face particular types of fear and control tactics, reports Dr. K. J. Wilson in her book *When Violence Begins at Home*. "One common type of intimidation is the threat of 'outing,' or the unwelcome disclosure of a person's sexual orientation," she says. "Batterers may threaten to 'out' their partners to family, friends, and employers. Depending on the circumstances, outing can mean loss of a job, support systems, and even child custody."[10]

Battered lesbians also face safety issues that differ from those of women with violent male partners. A batterer may try to enter the shelter or support group, claiming she is really the victim being battered, not the partner.

While in Denver I hired Robin, an exceptionally smart and qualified woman, as the Safehouse director of programs. She never spoke to me about her sexuality but I was certain she was a lesbian. After more than a year of consistently superb work, Robin's job performance deteriorated. She became somewhat erratic and emotional, coming in late, looking disheveled, and missing meetings and deadlines. One day I noted that her front tooth was broken. I asked her about the injury and told her I saw changes in her appearance and behavior and was concerned for her welfare. Robin, very distressed, told me that she had broken up with her girlfriend, Midge, and Midge hit her, breaking her tooth. Robin assured me she was taking appropriate measures and would be okay and safe. However, the next day Robin failed to come in to work or to call. Alarmed, I tried calling repeatedly and eventually drove to her house. Not finding her at home, I looked in the windows, tried the door, and finally left a note tucked under the front knocker telling her to call me immediately because I was worried about her. I said if I didn't hear from her I would call the police.

Robin called as soon as I returned to the office and told me she had gone into hiding because she was afraid of Midge, who continued to threaten and harass her. She asked if I could make sure that Midge was denied admission to the shelter if she tried to get in. Likewise for Midge's friends. They would seek "shelter" as a ruse to find her, Robin cautioned. Would I please tell the staff, most of whom reported directly to her, that she was a lesbian? She wanted them to know that she had left her partner, she had gone into hiding, and under no circumstances should any of them give Midge or her friends any information about Robin. The Safehouse staff, many of whom knew and liked Midge, were astonished and saddened by the revelations. They identified strategies for screening any "plants" Midge might try to get into the shelter and developed a comprehensive safety plan for Robin, their boss. None of us ever again doubted that one woman might hurt another.

Socioeconomic Factors

When I sought safety in a battered-women's shelter, I was the only one with a good job, a college degree, and a means of supporting myself. Over the years I discovered that my experience was typical. It is rare for a woman with resources and options to stay in a shelter unless, like me, she is in a seriously dangerous situation and requires the relative protection the shelter can provide. But I know battered women of every profession and socioeconomic class. They include high-level politicians and the wives of high-level politicians, doctors and doctors' wives, attorneys and attorneys' wives, television celebrities, and many others. The father of a dear friend was a university professor who shot and killed her mother, also a professional educator. My friend is now an attorney and a respected judge, helping to change the system so other children won't have to live through experiences similar to hers. Just like my friend's parents, many families are able to hide the violence behind expensive sunglasses and six-foot fences surrounding their acre-size lots. The women have cars to sleep in and credit cards to pay for counseling, and they find alternatives to shelter.

However, a disproportionate number of battered women and children are from families that are barely hanging on or have already fallen into the underclass of our society. While wife abuse is by no means confined to families living in poverty, studies of marital violence do support the hypothesis that it is more prone to occur in families lacking social and economic equity. The evidence is overwhelming that poverty is associated with a broad range of social problems, including higher birth rates in unwed mothers, teen pregnancy, crime and delinquency, drug-related problems, child maltreatment, higher rates of infant mortality, and various forms of violence, including rape and domestic violence.[11] Although the United States is in many ways one of the wealthiest nations in the world, rates of poverty in the United States exceed those of all similar countries.[12] In a cross-national analysis of poverty in eighteen developed nations, the US poverty rate of 17.8 percent was substantially higher than the rate of the others. The second-highest rate of poverty, in Italy, was 13.9 percent.[13] Within the United States, the highest rate of poverty is found among single mothers, some of whom are fleeing abusive relationships. Many women choose to stay in violent situations to avoid joining the ranks of poor single mothers.

Race and Ethnicity

Even more difficult to assess is the relationship between ethnicity and domestic violence, especially since people of color are disproportionately trapped in poverty. Women of color are also overrepresented in groups with poor education, limited job resources, language barriers, and fear of deportation. It is also likely that women of color are less likely to report abuse, particularly given the fact that reporting may result in separation from one's family and children, loss of livelihood, and perhaps forced deportation. Women of color are statistically more likely to become victims of domestic violence—but when comparing African American women and whites of similar income levels, levels of domestic violence are similar.[14]

According to the National Violence Against Women Survey, African American women experience higher rates of intimate-partner homicide when compared to white women.[15] An additional consideration regarding domestic abuse in African American communities is, of course, racism. An African American woman may be less likely to report her abuser or seek help because of fear of discrimination and the vulnerability of African American men to negative stereotyping and police brutality. The stereotyping isn't just relegated to African American men; black women also encounter stereotyping when seeking help. They have been portrayed as "domineering figures that require control." Most domestic-violence programs will probably support my observation that African American women are particularly susceptible to charges of "mutual" battering or of "inciting" the violence.

According to the National Violence Against Women Survey (NVAWS), there was little difference in Hispanic and non-Hispanic women's reports of intimate-partner violence,[16] a statistic that is hard for anyone who has worked in the field of domestic violence to reconcile with their experience. In one study, 48 percent of Hispanic women reported that their partner's violence against them increased after they immigrated to the United States.[17]

In my experience, Hispanics are often bound by the cultural traditions of "machismo," or excessive masculinity and a belief in conservative gender roles. It is unacceptable for a woman to be divorced, to marry several times, or to remain single. Religious beliefs may keep them from accessing birth control, resulting in large families, which can make it difficult for a family to move or to find affordable housing.

When a young Hispanic woman with twelve children came into the SafePlace shelter, I was struck by the sheer logistics of moving and caring for such a large brood. I wondered how she simply managed to get to the shelter with all twelve of her children. I was told that she and her children were transported to the shelter in a police van. But once at the shelter, public transportation was her only means of getting around — with, of course, all twelve of her children in tow. The logistics of transporting, clothing, bathing, feeding, and tending to twelve children, aged newborn to fourteen, practically ensured that she would stay with her husband. But the woman, an undocumented immigrant who spoke only fragmented English and had little education and no job skills, was finally faced with losing all of her children if she stayed with her husband. He was abusing the children as well as her. The family had to stay in the shelter for many months, as the mom worked with the staff to find affordable housing for such a large family, as well as some means of self-support.

Shelters are often overflowing with women of color and their children. The NVAWS also found a high incidence of domestic violence in Native American and Alaskan Indian women, as well as Asian and Pacific Islander women. A survey of immigrant Korean women found that a horrifying 60 percent had been battered by their husbands.[18] In Denver I met a Korean woman married to a US serviceman. Together, they had a seven-year-old son. Shelter staff members were stunned to learn that the Korean mother spoke no English, while her son spoke little Korean. Somehow, the father had further isolated his wife by restricting her communication with her son.

Additional Factors

As I have already noted, there is a strong relationship between domestic violence and substance abuse, on the part of both batterers and victims. In addition, family violence occurs most often among those under the age of thirty; the rate is more than double the rate for people between thirty-one and fifty.[19] Young mothers are also vulnerable; women who have children by age twenty-one are twice as likely to be victims of domestic violence as women of the same age who are not mothers.[20]

Imbalances in power and decision-making have also been found to feed domestic violence. Homes of families that hold traditional beliefs that women should be submissive to men are more likely to experience all types of family violence, including both child and spousal abuse. We often see this in the homes of ethnic minorities. Egalitarian households, in which decision-making is shared, are the least violent families, and homes in which all the decisions are made by either the wife or the husband have the highest rates of violence.[21]

❧

I have known victims of battering who fit all of the conventional patterns, and I have known victims who shatter all stereotypes. I have known victims who are rich and poor, old and young, straight and gay, male and female, people with disabilities and able-bodied. And I have seen these individuals overcome tremendous odds, then give back to help others. These women and men are no longer victims, and they are more than survivors — they have overcome enormous adversity and created lives of hope, determination, and joy. They have become heroes and role models for those around them.

6

survivors:
much more than
former victims

I am awed by the strength and resilience of survivors, and I am reminded that the people we work with are heroes.

—Julia Spann, SafePlace
Executive Director

W E HEAR A LOT ABOUT HEROES IN TODAY'S WORLD. BLOCK-
buster movies trumpet stories of superheroes with powers beyond imagination — heroes who when faced with overwhelming obstacles can rely on morphing into a monstrous green hulk, summoning
electrical storms to their defense, flying through the air, or activating
their X-ray vision. However, I know there are real heroes who walk
among us, people who have overcome astonishing odds without the benefit of superpowers, or even the things many of us take for granted: a good
education, a roof over our head, a job that pays a living wage, assistance
from supportive friends and family, a sound mind and body, access to affordable health care, access to a fair and just legal system, safe child care,
and the resilience and coping skills learned from a healthy childhood.
These are heroes who have been thrust into situations they haven't asked
for or been prepared for, but who have nevertheless overcome unbeliev-
able odds.

I have continued to work with battered-women's programs for decades because of the extraordinary survivors I have met along the way.
At dinner parties I am able to bring the room to total silence when responding to a question about my day. I am regularly asked how I can take
all the sadness. I can take the sadness because of the amazing successes
I see — unlikely heroes and astonishing acts of selflessness that help to
balance the grief. How many people have had the opportunity to do a job
where they could literally say they know they've helped to save people's
lives every day?

This chapter features the stories of just a few of the people I have
known who have transcended victimization to become much more than
former victims, or even survivors. These are the stories of heroes. Each
of these people has been able to take their personal tragedies and heart-
breaks and transform them into positive and powerful forces for good.
When tested, each took the sum of their lives lived thus far, their innate
gifts and strengths, and by continuing to live and grow and prosper became everyday heroes. Why is it that some with similar life stories become eternal victims, fragile, frightened ghosts of who they might have
been; others become raging, angry caricatures of their own abusers; and

still others effectively wall off their emotions, rejecting warmth and love while holding in pain and hurt. What special spark or experience allowed each of the remarkable people profiled in this chapter to dig deep and find uncommon resilience? I wish I had a definitive answer. I don't. But I do see common personality traits and characteristics among them.

Estrella Rochelli

Estrella Rochelli, a Latina with thick, dark hair and deep, brown eyes that sparkle with intelligence, was shot four times by her estranged husband as she ran from him down the side of a highway in Dallas. She was saved by a heroic couple who pulled her into their van as her husband stopped to reload his gun for the third time.

> *He said if I ever called the police he would kill me when he got out. He had found where I was living, but I was able to get away and hide in my sister's apartment. I called the police and they picked him up outside on the street as he was looking for me. I went to the police the next day and told them what he said he would do and begged them not to let him out of jail. The next morning—I remember it was a Monday—I told my sister that if I died I wanted her to make sure my organs were donated. I also remember smoking a cigarette, something I hadn't done in many years. Then I went to class and on to my job.*
>
> *I didn't know it but they had let him out of jail earlier that day. No one tried to notify me that he had been released. When I got off work at about nine that night, I went to my car and had pulled out of the parking lot and was waiting at a red light before I realized he was in a car behind me. Someone else was with him but we never found out who it was. He started shooting at my car so I took off through the red light and tried to get away, but I lost control and my car went up on a median and died. He was coming after me, shooting, and I couldn't get my car started, so I got out and started running. He shot me in the back and in my arm, but I didn't feel the bullets. I was zigzagging like you see in the movies.*

At one point the bullets stopped and I turned around and saw that he was reloading his gun. I remember standing about ten feet from him and being so mad! I wasn't scared, I just wanted to grab his gun and shoot him. Then I started begging for my life, begging for our daughters; I was the only one they had. He looked me in the eye and shot me again, this time in the neck. Then he shot me in the chest just above the heart, and I started running again.

I saw a van go by, and I tried to raise my hand to flag it down. I thought my arm was gone because I couldn't feel it, but when I touched it with my other arm I could tell it was still there. I thought they weren't going to stop, but then they came back and the woman pulled me into the back of the van. I remember she said, "Just get in." It was a man and a woman with one child and they owned a convenience store nearby. They took me there and were yelling for people to call the police and an ambulance.

My stomach was getting really big because it was filling up with blood, and I was so thirsty that I was begging for water. I heard one person say they shouldn't give me anything until the ambulance got there, then another woman said, "No, she's dying, just give her some water." The police and ambulance came and I told them to call my sister because my daughters were with her and I was afraid he would go after them next. I kept asking them to call my sister but they called my brother. My brother called my sister and made sure my girls were safe. They took me to Baylor Medical Center where everyone was standing outside waiting when the ambulance drove up. They rushed me into surgery, and I remember one woman's voice saying, "Don't worry about it. Everything will be okay." I don't know who it was but I held on to those words.

It took them a year to find and arrest my husband. At one point he talked to my sister and told her that he knew I had gone to Austin and that he was going to come down to Austin and "finish the job by putting a bullet in her brain." The FBI finally arrested him in Boston more than a year later.

Miraculously, Estrella suffered no permanent physical damage, and when released from the hospital she came to SafePlace with her three daughters. It wasn't safe for her to stay in Dallas because her husband had not yet been apprehended, and the SafePlace shelter was known for its extensive security features. By this time SafePlace was a large organization, employing well over a hundred people and helping thousands each year, so I rarely interacted individually with our clients. But I knew Estrella's dramatic story. Even today I feel a shiver when thinking of that heroic couple who put their lives at stake to help an unknown woman who was being attacked on the side of a highway.

Several years after Estrella had been in the shelter, I was introduced to the crowd at a March of Dimes fund-raising luncheon at the Four Seasons hotel. It was a typical banquet, with tables of eight or ten served an unremarkable chicken dinner by an efficient and nameless service staff. But this time, my waitress found me when the lunch was over. She said, "SafePlace saved my life. I just wanted to say thank you."

This was not an unusual occurrence; what was unusual was that when she started talking, I realized I knew this woman's story. This was Estrella, the woman who had very nearly died on a highway in Dallas. I stayed in touch with her and she became my friend. I once asked her if she knew that I had been in an abusive marriage prior to working at SafePlace. Her reaction affirmed my decision to tell these stories along with my own. She had no idea about my history and said, with surprise, "But you are white and educated." As I have said, I was lucky; I looked right, talked right, and had a good education and supportive friends and family. Estrella was not born lucky.

She was born in El Salvador, the second of eleven children, and came of age just as the civil war there was intensifying. From a very young age she woke up early to help with farm chores and then walked an hour to and from school, returning in late afternoon to work on the farm until dark. She had only one dress, which she washed out every night and hung to dry so it would be clean for her to wear the next day. She had no shoes until she was twelve or thirteen years old, and she would run quickly past the groups of boys so they wouldn't make fun of her bare feet. Her formal schooling in El Salvador ended when she completed the seventh grade.

When Estrella was sixteen, her parents became concerned that their daughter might be forced by one side or another to fight in the civil war, so they borrowed money from a friend in the United States, and Estrella flew to New York. Outside the airport terminal, she asked a group of young men if they knew where she could get a taxi. She spoke little English and had never been out of El Salvador. The men assured her they would help her, but then they pushed her into their car, holding her head down as they drove an hour out of the city. She said they were clearly intent on raping her at the very least. Thinking of the police dramas she had seen on television, she screamed at the men that her father was a police detective and would come after them. She was apparently believable because they stopped the car, pushed her out, and sped away. She found her way back to a place where she was able to call for a cab and make it to the home of her parent's friend.

Estrella was able to get her green card so she could work legally in the United States. She was hired as a waitress in a restaurant in New York. When she first met Pedro, a native of the Dominican Republic, he was working as lead chef in the restaurant where she waited tables. Her initial reaction to him was one of dislike. Much like my first opinion of Jay, she thought he was arrogant. But he pursued her aggressively and, alone and lonely in a strange country, Estrella eventually succumbed to his charms, marrying him and giving birth to three daughters. Their marriage was anything but happy. Pedro was insanely jealous and quickly became abusive toward Estrella, eventually precipitating her flight to Dallas.

From these experiences, Estrella has created a remarkable life. She has worked diligently to create a future for her daughters, who are astonishingly accomplished. They have attended private college preparatory schools on scholarship, and the oldest is now attending Princeton, again on a full scholarship. These are the young women whose father said would never amount to anything—he called them "dirt and whores, just like your mother."

Pedro was prosecuted for attempted murder and sentenced to a lengthy prison sentence. A month prior to his release date, he died in prison. No one in his family mourned his passing.

Estrella has moved into her own Habitat for Humanity home, and she works and continues to attend college part-time. Though she no longer lives under a cloud of fear from Pedro, she does continue to be challenged with struggles beyond those most of us experience. While working as a bartender at the Four Seasons, many of the tendons in her right hand were severed by a broken glass. She does physical therapy to regain range of movement and strength so she can continue with her work as a waitress and bartender, which pays a living wage. Recently, she went to the doctor because she was having a lot of pain in her neck. Following testing, the physician told her she had a small piece of metal lodged in her neck, a fragment of a bullet from Pedro's gun. Shortly thereafter, Estrella lost her Medicaid coverage due to state and federal budget cuts.

When asked what message she would give to other survivors of domestic abuse she says, "I love seeing a positive message for all the women who have the same or similar history as mine. I want to encourage them not to let that pain make them less or to think they cannot continue with their life. Mainly, I want to tell them to put all their effort into raising their kids, give all of their love to them, and tell themselves that their kids are the best reason they have to keep going no matter what. It is a miracle that I am still alive—do you see why I believe there is a God?"

Donna Stockton-Hicks

Donna, a former chair of the Austin SafePlace Board of Directors, along with her husband, Steve Hicks, has given millions of dollars over the past decade to assist those who need it most. Among their many community gifts was $1 million that they donated to SafePlace to build a child development center adjacent to the shelter facility. Her gift was prompted by the brutal death of the two-year-old daughter of a SafePlace client. The child's father had promised his estranged wife that he would "destroy her life." One day he picked up his daughter, Lucy, from her day care and flew with her to Haiti, his home country. He took Lucy to the home of his wife's mother and slit the baby's throat in front of the grandmother, who was meeting her granddaughter for the first time. I still question how a father could have carried his little girl on his lap from Austin to Haiti, knowing that he intended to kill her in such a brutal way. The father, the scion of a powerful Haitian family, was never prosecuted.

Blessed with a huge heart, Donna realized that she had the financial resources to help make other children safer. We at SafePlace had always known that children were vulnerable when in school or at day care—it is very difficult to keep a parent, even an abusive father, from accessing their children in these facilities. Yet children have to go to school, and mothers need care for their children while they work. One afternoon, the sorrow from Lucy's death still fresh and raw with all of us, Donna said to me, "Steve and I want to give SafePlace a million dollars, and we want you to use it to build a secure day-care center next to the shelter. No more Lucys."

Donna has the kind of ageless beauty that most of us yearn for. When she decided that she wanted to quit dying her hair and let it grow out to its natural silvery white, she shaved her head—and she looked fabulous! She lives in a mansion and owns vacation homes around the country. She and her husband, a kind and gentle man who absolutely adores her, have the wherewithal and the inclination to help those who haven't been so blessed.

Her life has not always been so good. She shares her personal story so others can see that even the rich and powerful have sometimes lived with inner shame, doubt, and self-blame, and have survived victimization. Born in Fort Worth, Texas, Donna, the youngest of three children, was named for the Madonna. Her father was a well-known and respected community leader who founded a large accounting firm, served as the chair of the local United Way Campaign, and helped to establish the Women's Center, an agency providing sexual-abuse and rape-crisis prevention and intervention services, as well as other programs to empower and assist women and children. He worked long hours and was rarely home to assist his wife, a stay-at-home mom who, Donna says, was overwhelmed with raising three children alone and usually slept for several hours during the afternoon. Only as an adult did Donna realize that her mother was self-medicating through the use of tranquilizers. Her parents were completely engaged in the Church of Christ, which preached a fundamentalist doctrine delineating rigid gender roles, a system of beliefs that Donna rebelled against from an early age.

As a preadolescent, Donna's primary relationship was with her brother, who was five years older. He bought her nice gifts, including her first pair of roller skates and a Barbie doll. He also critiqued her wardrobe, telling her what she could and could not wear, monitored her friends, and often acted more like a boyfriend than a brother. She remembers feeling as though her brother really loved her. Unfortunately, he also sexually abused her. Her very first memories are of him fondling her between her legs when she was five years old. The abuse continued until she was in middle school and her brother went to college and then to Vietnam.

When Donna was twenty-five and divorced with two children, she and her brother were both home for a family event and sleeping on separate couches in the living room. As she was falling asleep her brother asked, "Are you awake?"

"Yes," said Donna.

"I'm going to come over and touch you," he whispered.

Donna got up and left the room, going to her sleeping children. Climbing into bed between her tiny son and daughter, Donna said she knew that she was escaping to them for safety. She hoped that their two little bodies could protect her from her brother's attentions.

Donna had left home at eighteen to marry a Navy pilot four years her senior. She was married to him for seven years, and they had two children—a daughter, Shelley, and a son, Jason. She also completed two years of college. Following the end of her marriage she became involved with a man named B.J. She was attracted to his "bad-boy charm" and remembers him as having "all the right moves." He would also slap her and abuse her verbally—behavior that quickly escalated to life-threatening attacks, which sometimes occurred in front of her children, now ages six and three.

The end of the relationship was precipitated by an attack at a lake on what was supposed to be a fun weekend outing. B.J. was drunk on scotch and, as was often the case when he drank, his anger toward Donna escalated. He grabbed Donna by her hair and pushed her head underwater, holding her down until she thought her lungs would burst. He finally pulled her head out of the water by her hair, backhanded her across the face, and yelled at her, "You're a fucking whore." He pushed her head back underwater. He was finally brought to his senses, and stopped the attack, by the screams and pleas of Donna's children. "Yes, the screaming of my two children got his attention," she says. "That was the last day I ever spent with him." When B.J. passed out from drinking, Donna got her kids and left for her parents' home.

B.J., however, didn't give up easily. He and Donna's brother were drinking buddies, and the family believed B.J.'s version of events. He successfully enlisted them in trying to convince her she should return to the relationship. Because of their advocacy for B.J., Donna finally saw that she could not look to her family for safety. She fled the state, moving with her kids to Louisiana. She was a young, divorced mother whose parents had turned away from her, she was living in a state apart from everyone she knew, her credit was ruined because B.J. had run up all of her credit cards, and she had no means of financial support.

Donna soon met a man several years her senior and married him quickly. She says, "I think my self-esteem was so low and I felt so powerless to take care of those two children that I looked to the first man who 'talked the talk' and promised me he would take care of us. He showed sympathy to me for previous trauma. It was just such a relief at first to hand over my life. Quite frankly, I was so numb at that point, and so beaten down, I didn't spend much time thinking about it."

She stayed in the marriage for eleven years. But once again she found herself in a relationship with a man who drank too much. Donna says, "He was a lovely man as long as I was his little girl who minded." Breaking out of that role, one she'd learned from childhood, has been one of the hardest lessons for Donna to learn, and she credits much of her personal growth to Al-Anon, years of therapy, and the support of Steve, her husband for the last fifteen years. She attributes her therapist, Linda, with changing her life: "She never gave up on me and seldom showed any surprise as, through the years, I unraveled my story. I really owe my sanity to her." She continues, "What I have learned is that my whole idea of love from a man was about sex and violence. I had a total lack of respect for myself. My therapist and Al-Anon helped me to understand why I would keep choosing men who verbally berated me and treated me awful. The theme of all these men was addiction to alcohol. I didn't know it at the time, but each and every man I chose was an alcoholic."

Donna's current husband, Steve, is a recovering alcoholic and a spokesperson for and supporter of programs addressing issues of addiction. Their partnership has helped Donna rebuild her life and heal from the trauma of her earlier years. Together they have made a fortune, first in radio and later in real estate and other investments. Most important, Steve has always believed in Donna and supported her as she has made her journey from victim to survivor to helper and hero. About her generous philanthropy she says, "I used to think that I made these gifts in order to make up, in some small way, for the unsafe circumstances I put my kids in when they were young. Now I realize that, through my gifts, I have also been trying to heal myself—the little five-year-old child that no one was there for."

Donna eventually confronted her brother about the childhood sexual abuse. He told their parents that Donna was on drugs and making absurd allegations against him. Her father tried calling her therapist, who appropriately refused to speak to him. The therapist told Donna, "In your family, you have been set up to be the crazy one."

Donna's mother responded to the allegations by saying, "Can't you just get over this? You are tearing our family apart." Donna replied, "Mom, you can have a relationship with your son and you can have a relationship with your daughter, but I will not have a relationship with my perpetrator."

Donna's mother eventually reconciled herself to having separate relationships with her children, but she never again spoke of the matter. Many years later, after the death of her mother, Donna's sister found a years-old letter written from her aunt to their mother that said, "I will never come to your house again. It was just too hard to watch the abuse that your son was doing to your daughter. It was all I could do not to snatch Donna up and get her out of that house." Donna says that her aunt and her mother were estranged thereafter.

As is the case in my own family, Donna has been able to track abuse through more than one generation of her family. Donna's mother, Mozelle, spoke to her once of her own history of sexual abuse. Mozelle's father was killed in a cotton gin accident when his two daughters were quite young. Mozelle's mother, Marjorie, remarried and had another child, a son. Her new husband sexually abused his two stepdaughters, and Marjorie was desperate to get the girls away from him. Her husband said, "I'll give you a divorce and you can have your girls, but you'll never see your son again." She got the divorce and he was true to his word; Marjorie never again saw her son. Donna's mother had no memory of her brother.

As with my family, Donna wasn't made privy to this history of familial abuse until after she had already experienced sexual and domestic violence herself. Still, the abuse, even though it was never spoken of, affected later generations. It has stopped with Donna. In addition, she has worked hard through her charitable work to ensure safety for many generations of families — most of whom she will never meet or know.

Ed Born-Long

One of my favorite stories about Ed is how he came by his last name. Ed Born met Chris Long, his wife of twenty-five years, at a meeting for "tall singles." They fell in love, got married, and blended their names to become Ed and Chris Born-Long.

I first met Ed, a big, rumpled man with sad blue eyes, hound-dog jowls, and an infectious grin, when he walked into our office with a thousand-dollar check in hand. Our office was temporarily located in the Brackenridge Hospital Administrative building while we were raising money to build a new resource center. The check was a donation from the Central Texas Roofing Contractors Association, of which Ed was president, and the contribution was being made in memory of his daughter, Annie, who had recently been brutally murdered. Ed also wanted to volunteer. "I don't know how I can help," he said. "I'm just an old roofer. But

I have to do something to keep this from happening to someone else's daughter."

Ed, who had just returned from burying Annie in California, knew that reaching out to assist others would help him to heal. He says, "When I first went into SafePlace, I could hardly talk. I had tears in my eyes. They invited me in. It was a tiny office and they were going over some financial stuff, and they put it aside and made time for me. Everyone was taken by how soon after the whole thing this was. Kelly put me in touch with a lot of people and gave me work to do — that's how I got through."

Immediately after his daughter's murder, Ed traveled to the California mountains. He says:

> *I went up to Lake Tahoe. You can imagine places like that; you know you're right next to God up there. I had questions: What do I really believe in? How do I see this? And what are my motives going to be? Because I didn't know. What I decided by lying up in the mountains for two days, just thinking, was that I was going to be positive. Whatever happened, I decided I was going to choose the positive way each time. I didn't care what was going to happen to this guy. That's his crime. What I was going to do was remember my daughter well and go positive from there.*

Ed's daughter, Andrea Mercedes Born, was eleven days short of her twenty-first birthday on 4 July 1997, when she was shot twice in the head, execution style. Her body was set on fire in an orchard in Madera County, California. Her remains were found by the side of the road, requiring identification through dental records. Rather than a celebratory event, Annie's twenty-first birthday was marked by her cremation and a memorial service commemorating her life. Three years passed before the killer, Annie's abusive ex-boyfriend, was brought to justice and sentenced to fifteen years to life for her murder. Yet in those three years, and afterward, Ed's decision to stay positive despite his great loss would be an enormous boon for SafePlace and would help many others.

Andrea, who had blonde curls and a gentle smile, was working two jobs to pay her way through college at Fresno State University. She had starred in several community-theatre productions and wrote poetry that she kept in a journal by her bed. Annie was last seen in the company of her former boyfriend, a relationship that was known for being abusive and from which she was trying to extricate herself. Despite the evidence, the former boyfriend wasn't arrested right away, and Ed and his former wife, Gloria Barnes, Annie's mother, will tell you the investigation was badly bungled. After the first few months it was relegated to the cold-case files, but Gloria, who worked as a clerk with the Madera County court system, continued to agitate for an arrest. Her campaign ultimately resulted in Annie's murder being featured on a televised episode of *Crime Stoppers* and a fifty-thousand-dollar reward being offered.

A billboard was rented for a week on a major highway to publicize the reward. Annie's mother stood beneath that billboard for the entire week in order to generate attention for the murder and the potential reward. Eventually, her tenacity paid off. Three years after the murder, Jacob Lee Travis was arrested for first-degree murder. In his statement to the judge, Travis wrote that he loved Annie so much, he didn't want to see her with someone else. If he couldn't have her, he wrote, no one could.

On 7 March 2003 Travis pled guilty to second-degree murder and was sentenced to serve fifteen years to life. Annie's friends and family were distressed that the man who murdered their loved one might be a free man after only eleven years, including credit for time already served. Many sent letters of grief and outrage, believing that Travis should stay behind bars for the rest of his life. Ed and Gloria are committed to actively tracking future court proceedings and advocating for Travis' continued imprisonment.

"When Annie was first dead, life looked to me like a big, big black hole," Ed said. He chose to channel his grief and rage into helping Safe-Place. He persuaded the Central Texas Roofing Contractors, as well as multiple roofing suppliers, to perform a pro-bono roofing job for Safe-Place's new resource center, which saved the organization over a hundred thousand dollars in construction costs. Just after dawn on a Saturday morning, pickup trucks carrying hundreds of brawny roofers converged on the site with tools, materials, and Artz Rib House barbeque in hand.

Every major media outlet covered this enormous outpouring of generosity from roofing contractors in support of their friend and colleague.

"It was like a snowball going downhill," Ed said. "As word got around, a lot of my friends and the roof contractors — many of whom I knew because I was president of the association — they all got together and said they wanted to donate the labor for the new resource center. Different people heard about it; the manufacturers chipped in the membrane. We had a meeting over at Artz Rib House, and Art overheard and said he wanted to donate the food. A consulting agency said there wasn't anything left for them to do, so they did the beverages. It was just magical."

Ed and his wife, Chris, also became involved with the SafePlace Walk for Safe Families, an annual fund-raising event that relied on teams and pledges to raise hundreds of thousands of dollars to support the general operating funds of the organization. "Annie's Team," organized by Ed, Chris, and his many friends, always raised the most money and generated the most walkers. He also stepped forward as a spokesperson, saying, "If they wanted me to go on TV and do spots to help promote the walk, why not? I've already paid the highest price."

Annie wasn't the first daughter Ed had lost. Much earlier he had given up parental rights to an older daughter, Emilie. In the late sixties he'd married a "hippie girl." They moved to Europe and adopted a carefree lifestyle. They had Emilie, but decided to go their separate ways. Emilie's mother remarried and settled down. Ed says, "They gave me the papers and asked me to sign 'em so that the new husband could adopt Emilie and they'd be a family, and then they wouldn't chase me for child support. I didn't have a better program than that, so I finally signed those papers after first tearing them up."

Ed and Annie were searching for Emilie prior to Annie's death. Annie wanted to meet her sister. Following Annie's death, Emilie actually found Ed, who now delights in his role as a father and grandfather. Annie can never be replaced in Ed's heart, but his heart is as big as Texas — it has plenty of room for his wife, Annie, Emilie, Emilie's four children, and SafePlace.

Kimberly Wisseman

All too often, the people who devote their lives to creating safe and peaceful homes and communities are, like me, the same people who have benefited from the work of those who came before them. One such person is Kimberly Wisseman, a lovely, kind, smart, and dedicated woman with long, white-blond hair and a slender build. She holds a master's degree in social work from California State University in Long Beach and is a compassionate and talented counselor of people who have been victimized by violence. She has been married to Phil, a handsome engineer with a gentle demeanor, for nine years, and together they have a five-year-old son, Evan, the spitting image of his mother but with his father's big brown eyes.

Kimberly has used a wheelchair for mobility for the past twenty-five years because of a car accident at the age of sixteen. The accident left her with a spinal cord injury that caused paralysis from the neck down. Since then, Kimberly has required assistance to help with the most basic activities of bathing, dressing, toileting, and getting out of bed in the morning.

Kimberly is also a survivor of domestic violence, sexual assault, and stalking. She has been victimized repeatedly, both by a man who said he loved her and by strangers. For years Kimberly has courageously told her story of vulnerability, survival, courage, and resilience to audiences across the country. She has done more than most of us could imagine in order to educate others about violence against people with disabilities. A SafePlace counselor from 1998 through 2007, she was honored in 2002 with the Special Courage Award by the US Department of Justice, Office for Victims of Crime.

Kimberly didn't begin life thinking she would be a role model and an inspiration. She was reared as an only child. When she was ten, her parents divorced and she stayed with her mother in Hawaii. A few years later, she decided to move to Texas to live with her aunt and uncle. She attended West Lake High School, in Austin, where she was trying out for the drill team just before her accident.

Kimberly credits a part of her resilience to the fact that she experienced significant health and family challenges while still a young child.

She endured three major surgeries at age six, one of which resulted in a near-death experience. She vividly recalls "sitting on a file cabinet above the fray, watching the doctors and nurses trying to bring me back to life." She also learned at a young age to make decisions for herself. After her parent's divorce, she had to make decisions that guided her life, including where she would live and go to school, and how she would interact with her parents.

After the accident, Kimberly says she found herself fighting for her life: "The doctors told me that if I lived through the surgery I would never walk again, never get married, never have children, and I would live the life of a vegetable. I contemplated suicide and decided that if I was going to live, I wanted to live my life the way I was planning before I became disabled. So, scared to death, I ventured off to college."

As a senior at Texas A&M, recently broken up with a boyfriend from high school, she began dating Juan. "He had pursued me aggressively, showing up on campus wherever I was and constantly asking me to go out with him," she says. "Our first several months together were wonderful, and when, after six months, he wanted to move in together, I said yes. Because of my disability I require attendant-care services, so I thought this was a great idea."

After they set up housekeeping, Juan became controlling and jealous. If she came home late from class, he wanted to know where she had been. If he saw her talking to someone, he would get angry. "We started arguing a lot, and he would throw things around our apartment," she remembers. "Then he said that he wanted to get married. I felt that we were too young and had only been together a short time. So he proposed marriage to me in front of a group of our friends, making me feel too uncomfortable to say no." After the two became engaged, Juan began referring to Kimberly as his "pretty bird in a cage," and the verbal and emotional abuse rapidly escalated into physical violence, each episode worse than the one before.

"One day I was sitting on the floor and we were arguing," she says. "He took off all my clothes and watched as I was crying and trying to scoot my body to the telephone to call for help. Another day when I came home late from class, he was sitting on the couch with a butcher knife in his hand. He grabbed me by my feet and pulled me out of the wheelchair, climbed on top of me, and started stabbing the knife on the floor around my head and choking me. After that incident, I realized I wanted out of the relationship."

Shortly thereafter, Kimberly and Juan were driving in the car and Kimberly suggested they spend some time apart. Juan pulled over and stopped the car, got out, walked around to the passenger side, picked Kimberly up, and set her down on the side of the road. He got back in the car and drove off about a half a block, then put the car in reverse and sped back to Kimberly, stopping only feet in front of her and causing gravel to fly around her. "He put me back in the car and I started to take off my engagement ring," Kimberly says. "He grabbed my wrist and bent my arm completely backwards until we heard it break. He said, 'If I can't have you, no one can.'"

Juan took Kimberly to the emergency room, where he never left her side. No one in the hospital ever tried to separate the two to ask how her arm had been broken. "He said he would kill me if I told, so I think I just said I had fallen," Kimberly recalls. "I knew my life was in danger and I knew I wanted out of this relationship. But I only had three months left until graduation and I thought, 'If this is the man who loves me, and he's doing these things to me, what would someone else do to me, someone that I hired and brought into my home to provide attendant-care services?' That idea felt scarier to me. So I thought I could manage this relationship for three more months."

One night Juan kept Kimberly up all night, cutting her wrists a little and telling her, "If you leave me, I'll make sure we both die." She says, "I had learned how to de-escalate the arguments. If I would say, 'Yes, it's my fault, yes, I'm sorry, yes, I'll marry you,' and then we would have sex, he would stop hurting me, and the argument would be over and everything would be fine."

Three weeks later, she was admitted to the hospital with a broken nose, bites on her face, broken ribs, and a permanently damaged sternum. Juan was arrested and charged with two counts of aggravated assault with a deadly weapon and serious bodily injury. "About a year later the trial started, and on the witness stand I was portrayed by the defending attorney as a woman with a severe disability whom no man would ever want or ever love, and how wonderful his client was for giving up his life to take care of me," Kimberly says. "The broken bones that I sustained were explained by saying apparently I just fell out of my wheelchair a lot."

Juan's former girlfriend came to court and testified about the abuse she had endured, abuse that was in many ways almost identical to what Kimberly experienced. She testified to his holding her down on the bed and stabbing around her head with a butcher knife. She said she saved the sheet with the knife holes in it so she would be reminded what he was like if she considered returning to him.

Despite the testimony from physicians, police, his former victim, the evidence of the rug with stab marks, and a butcher knife with a bent tip, Juan was found not guilty.

"I felt completely revictimized, only this time by the system," Kimberly says. "I remember that one of the jurors was a female emergency room nurse. I thought, 'If she can't believe me, how might it be for others who come into the emergency room?' "

The prosecuting attorneys were determined that Juan should pay for his crimes, so they filed charges on a lesser charge. When the second trial started a few months later, Kimberly didn't feel emotionally strong enough to go through the ordeal again, so the state proceeded without her. Juan pleaded no contest and was sentenced to two years' probation and psychiatric counseling. He didn't even have to do the counseling unless he "didn't have to incur any expense." He had to pay $629 in court costs.

"That didn't feel like any justice," Kimberly remembers. "He was, however, kicked out of Texas A&M University permanently. It was a very small victory for me."

Kimberly got on with her life and moved to California to attend graduate school. She also met and began dating the man who is now her husband, Phil, at a gathering for University of Texas and Texas A&M

alumni who lived in California. Though they rooted for opposite teams, they hit it off.

"One Friday evening, shortly after I graduated with my master's degree, my attendant and I were at home," Kimberly says. "I had just hung up the phone from talking to my mother when I heard a noise in my bedroom. I called for my attendant to come out and see what the noise was. About that time we saw two men walking out of my bedroom. They had come in through my bedroom window. One had a gun and one had a knife. The men pushed my attendant at gunpoint back into her room, threw a mattress over her, and robbed her. The other man opened up the sliding glass door and in walked two more men. I was then robbed and raped."

One man held a knife to Kimberly's throat and another a gun to her head as they sexually assaulted her and took everything of value in the apartment. Toward the end of the assault, they told her they had been watching her and had "picked" her.

"Before they left they told me that if the police got them they would come back for me," Kimberly remembers. "So my attendant and I waited the ten minutes they had specified before going into the parking lot and trying to contact someone to help us. Some neighbors came out, and the security guard drove up. I was taken to the hospital and given a rape exam and there was an investigation. There were never any criminal charges, because those four men have never been found." Phil slept on Kimberly's couch for two weeks after the incident.

Kimberly filed a civil suit against the security company and the apartment complex, because the security guard was never around throughout the assault. "During the investigation," Kimberly says, "the attorneys for the security company asked me questions such as, 'You're paralyzed, so how do you know you were raped?' And, 'If you can't feel anything, how do you know you were penetrated?' Those questions humiliated me and made me feel devalued. Because of that I chose to settle out of court, once again feeling victimized by the system. I realized that as a woman with a disability I am seen as an easy target."

Soon thereafter, Kimberly moved back to Texas. It took Phil two more years to find a job in Austin so he could join her.

Kimberly says that looking back on her relationship with Juan, she never thought of a shelter as an option. That was right at the time of the passage of the Americans with Disabilities Act, and most buildings, even those housing basic community services and businesses such as restaurants, were generally not accessible to her. She says that if she had received education on domestic violence and information on safety planning, and had had an accessible shelter, she would have had options to get out of that relationship before she was severely beaten.

"In 1996, after the sexual assault, I did receive services from a rape crisis center, and those services were critical in my recovery process," Kimberly says. "Because of those services I am no longer a victim. I am a survivor."

When asked what message is most important to convey, Kimberly says she wants people to understand the vulnerability of people with disabilities, vulnerabilities beyond what most of us can imagine. She continues to face challenges every day that would leave many of us weeping in self-pity. Kimberly and Phil get up at 5:45 AM every morning, after already waking up several times during the night so he can help her to turn over and empty her catheter. They have a live-in attendant Monday through Friday, who gets up at 7:00 AM. By 8:30 AM their son, Evan, is at school and Phil is at work, and Kimberly and her attendant manage the rest of the day until Kimberly picks Evan up from school. By the time Phil arrives home from work, the attendant has ended her workday and retired to her bedroom, and Phil and Kimberly prepare dinner, get Evan ready for bed, and have the slice of adult alone time that all parents covet.

When they married, all governmental financial assistance for Kimberly ceased; they currently spend more than $25,000 a year in out-of-pocket expenses just to pay for the basics of managing Kimberly's disability. Her health care is covered by Phil's medical insurance through his job with AT&T, leaving them — even more than most — worried about what might happen if he lost his job. While she was still working, the Texas Department of Assistive and Rehabilitative Services (TDARS) helped to pay for expenses, such as her motorized wheelchair and the adapted van that allows her to drive independently.

Even if she returned to work, at age forty-one, Kimberly has already reached her lifetime maximum allowable payout from TDARS. Phil pays the attendant out of his paycheck. As Kimberly puts it, "It costs us $3,000 a year just for me to pee." The family absorbs the cost of intermittent catheterization and of all other expenses. The replacement cost for her wheelchairs, which last about five years, is $15,000; a new van would cost $100,000.

"I have been through horrible challenges and experiences, but I have a beautiful life today, a wonderful husband and child," Kimberly says. "Through each of my experiences I have gotten stronger, and at the root of that has been my faith in God. Through each challenge I have asked God to see me through, and each time I have seen how He has answered my prayers and it has made me stronger. It has strengthened my faith to know to trust in Him to get through whatever challenges I have faced and continue to face."

I can still vividly remember the day Kimberly told me she was pregnant. We were in the reception area at SafePlace, and she patted her very slightly rounded tummy and told me she was having a baby, a son that she and Phil prayed and fought for. It wasn't easy for someone with Kimberly's disability to carry a pregnancy to term, but Kimberly has never taken the easy route through life.

She fights back tears as she talks about how hard it is not to be able to run and play with her son in the way they both want, and to push him in a swing. But in her usual can-do fashion, Kimberly has figured out other ways to play with him. She says she can put her wheelchair into high gear and keep up with him on his bike, and though she may not be able to lift her arms to throw a basketball, she is darn good at blocking the ball. They love tickle fights and wrestling. She has found toys he can play with independently or that she can enjoy with him. In being a mother — as in everything else — Kimberly doesn't give up.

Kimberly Wisseman is a hero to thousands who have worked with her, been counseled by her, and heard her speak. And she is a hero to the husband and son who love her and think of her as a beautiful, smart, sexy, nurturing, sassy wife and mother. She has shown others with and without disabilities how to live their lives on their own terms, never fearing to grab for the brass ring.

Thomasina Tijerina

Every day, at least once, I think, "I love my husband!" Since I'm a relative newlywed, people are still asking, "How's married life?" When I say, "It's great!" I know they're wondering when it'll change or thinking, "Just wait." Well, I didn't say I don't get angry with him or that he's 100 percent perfect 100 percent of the time. I'm just saying that for the most part it's great most of the time. I'm totally smitten with my husband. I know that should wear off after a while—but I hope not for a long, long time, if ever.

I experienced relationships, and a marriage, where it wasn't equal; it wasn't great. One person gave too much or didn't give enough; it was never balanced. Anger, fear, depression, sadness, regret, frustration, guilt—not just sometimes, but constant unhappiness was the predominant feeling I had in those relationships. So I have experienced the worst of the worst and now I'm being blessed with the best of the best.

I hope my daughters, my sisters, my friends, and any women who have not yet experienced their own best of the best, and are feeling that they may never do so, will someday come to know the feelings I have every day. Life's good. Strive to be healthy and happy—even when you're sick or unhappy. The goal is to be happy. Keep the faith.

Feel free to share this with anyone who might need a little encouragement. They need to know that things can, and usually do, get better.

Thomasina asked that I tell her story backward. She wanted me to start from February 2009, the day we sat down to talk. She is madly in love with her second husband, Daniel. She has four grown daughters, three currently in college, all doing well. She has a secure, good-paying job as manager of a department of the Division of Worker's Compensation for the Texas Department of Insurance, with sixteen employees reporting to her. And she is proud to be a role model and helper for others working to overcome hardship. I am most struck by her ability to rise above the overwhelming adversity in her life, to see the patterns and dead ends in her past, and to chart a new course filled with peace and hope.

A light-skinned African American woman who originally hales from South Carolina, she arrived for lunch dressed in a brilliant red sweater and blue jeans. She told me she has been working to get her personal trainer certification and is focusing on fitness, as opposed to weight reduction. It shows — she could easily pass for a decade younger than her fifty years. Six months ago she married Daniel, an accountant who also works for the state of Texas. They met when both worked as temporaries in the same office. She said he would often come back to talk to the people working in her area and she thought he was a really nice guy. A woman sitting next to her finally said, "I think he's sweet on you."

"No, he talks to everyone."

"I don't think so. He has to go right past me to get to you, and I don't see him stopping at my desk."

Daniel and Thomasina worked together on a project in the file room, and she loved that they laughed. From the beginning they had a good time together.

Daniel's wife had died from colon cancer four years earlier, leaving him with two young, grieving children to rear alone while coping with his own loss and grief. Thomasina and Daniel had both experienced enormous hardship. Having gone through hard times separately, they recognize what is truly important and appreciate the happiness they have found with each other.

Thomasina was born and reared in the still segregated Deep South. Her light skin color set her apart from the others in her family and her school. The other African American kids didn't accept her because she was too "white," and the whites didn't accept her because she was "black."

In all the years I have known Thomasina, I have never once heard her convey any sense of being judged because of the color of her skin, but as I listened to her story it was clear that at times she was victimized because of stereotyping and racism.

Her stepfather began sexually abusing her at such a young age that she can't even remember when it wasn't happening. Until the age of twelve she thought he was her biological father. She later learned that her mother was pregnant by someone else when she married the step-father. Her stepfather's family was very poor, but her mother was from a relatively affluent family that owned land and lived comfortably com-pared to most around them. Thomasina believes her mother's family was embarrassed at having an unmarried pregnant daughter and may even have paid her stepfather's family to arrange the marriage. They went on to have children together, two sons. Thomasina believes the fact that they were her stepfather's biological children helped to exempt them from the sexual abuse he perpetrated against her.

Sexual abuse of a young child is the ultimate betrayal, particularly when the child seeks protection and her or his efforts are rebuffed. Thomasina told her mother of her stepfather's abuse, and her mother, doubting her words, took her to a physician for a physical exam. The doctor said the exam was inconclusive, so her mother returned home, choosing to believe in her husband and to disbelieve Thomasina's claims.

Like many incest survivors, Thomasina says she started to act out sexually at a young age. When she was only twelve years old she decided to have sex with her fifteen-year-old neighbor, whom she considered her boyfriend. A few days after their first sexual encounter, the boy called and asked her to come over. They ended up having sex again, which she emphasizes was voluntary. But when they were finished, four of his friends came into the room. The five boys took turns holding her down while the others raped her. The boys did not consider their actions rape. Her supposed boyfriend acted as though they had a right to do what they did. He said simply and unapologetically, "We pulled a train on you," as if it were the same kind of thing as tying a can to the tail of a cat—sort of unkind, but "what boys do."

Thomasina told no one. She had already tried "telling" on her stepfather, and she hadn't been believed. She later tried to end her own life. She was almost successful and credits the near-death experience that ensued with giving her the optimism that infuses her personality today.

At the age of thirteen, Thomasina was again raped. She was at school and was assaulted by a fellow student while on her way to P.E. When she finally stumbled, hysterical, into the gym, her teacher convinced her to go with her to the principal's office. In her hysteria she began to confuse the traumas of her short life, repeatedly saying to the principal, "My stepfather will be so mad that I let another man touch me."

Finally, someone began to see that something was very wrong in Thomasina's household. However, no arrest was made because the police said she had initially given conflicting statements. Furthermore, she was taken to the same doctor who had refused to confirm her stepfather's sexual abuse. This time he told Thomasina's mother that she "was raped because she had on a brown polka-dot miniskirt and was asking for it." A part of Thomasina began to believe that she had brought these things on herself.

When I asked directly, Thomasina admitted that she is certain the physician, an older white Southern man, held opinions that were influenced by racism and stereotyping. From these incidents she learned to be wary and mistrustful of law enforcement, doctors, and her own family.

Following the school rape she was sent to stay with her mother's parents. Her mother continued living with her stepfather, and Thomasina was not allowed to return home as long as they were together. However, her acting out escalated, and she became difficult for her grandparents to control. Eventually her mother came to take her back home. However, her stepfather had told Thomasina he would kill her if she tried to come home. Terrified of his threats and of the possibility of returning to the abusive environment, Thomasina ran away. By this time her mother had made the stepfather leave the house, but he lived right next door.

Thomasina went to college at Lander University, just twenty-five miles from her home. She remembers her college years as fun, but even then she found herself involved in unhealthy relationships. The boyfriend she had during her freshman year slapped her when he found out a previous boyfriend had called her on the phone. "The funny thing is," she says, "the former boyfriend was calling to tell me he was getting married. There was nothing between us. He was just a friend." She was surprised to see such jealousy and rage over an innocent incident and broke up with her boyfriend for good.

Thomasina then became involved with a married man. She tried to break if off with him several times, and each time he became extremely volatile, stalking her and threatening any other men she spoke with. The relationship was finally terminated when she graduated from college and moved to Houston.

Almost unbelievably, except to those who have studied the phenomenon of revictimization, Thomasina was raped yet again while living in Houston. While waiting outside for a ride to take her to work, a man held a knife to her back, pushed her into a vacant building, and brutally assaulted her. Not trusting the police or doctors, she sought neither medical care nor police intervention.

Research shows that women who have been raped previously are at greater risk of being raped again and that being the victim of child sexual abuse doubles the likelihood of adult sexual victimization.[1] Like Thomasina, women and men who are repeatedly victimized have often failed to learn good coping and self-protection skills when young; they haven't learned how to interpret the signals a predator sends out. They may live in unsafe neighborhoods or with family and friends who are prone to violence.

Shortly after the sexual assault Thomasina moved in with a man who told her he would protect her. She became pregnant. He became abusive toward her, and she ended the relationship when she was five months pregnant, moving into an apartment on her own. About a year later, as a single working mom with a seven-month-old daughter, she met her first husband, Jackson. They met in the laundry room and she remembers that he was nice to both her and her baby girl and she liked his freckles. She thought he was cute. He was good to her in the beginning, but the relationship moved very quickly. They met in July and were married in

September. Even the day they married Thomasina knew she didn't really love him, but she wanted to give her baby the stability of a home with a mother and father.

Jackson, who was from Nigeria, was in the United States going to school. His father had three wives, and he came from a culture that elevated men over women and in which sons held a position of entitlement. But his and Thomasina's marriage was good for many years. Together they moved to Denton, Texas, so Thomasina could pursue her master's degree in library sciences. They had three more daughters and built two successful businesses, a nightclub and a pizza parlor. However, Thomasina became ill, at times needing to use a wheelchair for mobility, and her diagnosis and prognosis weren't at all clear. For a time the doctors thought she had multiple sclerosis, but as her symptoms abated they began to question the diagnosis. Eventually the family decided to move to Austin so she could get better care. Though she still experiences very erratic and periodic lapses in her health, no clear diagnosis has ever been made.

The marriage began to deteriorate rapidly once they were in Austin. Thomasina worked and took care of the four girls, while Jackson, whose businesses had failed, refused to even look for a job. Later she found out that he had become involved with one of the infamous Nigerian bank and mail-fraud schemes. When Thomasina lost her job, the entire family of six was forced to live on her meager unemployment benefits.

Jackson was abusive and Thomasina called the SafePlace shelter but, as was so often the case, the shelter was full. Upon talking with the crisis-line staff, it was determined that she was not in immediate danger. They talked about safety planning, and Thomasina and her girls were placed on a waiting list. Thomasina, judging that her case wasn't urgent enough, said she would have felt guilty taking a bed away from someone who might be in more immediate danger. This sequence of events reinforced Thomasina's reluctance to make waves or cause trouble; she didn't make another call to ask for shelter.

The situation at her home continued to deteriorate. On a Sunday afternoon she called a mutual friend in South Carolina. At the end of the conversation the friend, who was male, said, "Tell Jackson 'hi' from me."

Jackson, who had been listening to the whole conversation on an extension in another room, said, "You don't have to tell me anything — I've been listening to the whole call." He flew into a rage, screaming and yelling, questioning his daughter's paternity in front of Thomasina and her daughter, and beating Thomasina, who fled to her daughters' room until Jackson fell asleep a few hours later. Thomasina snuck out of the house and ran to a nearby 7-11, where she called the police. The police picked her up at the convenience store, looked at her bruises, listened to her story, and took her back to her house to get her daughters and a few personal belongings. The police then transported her and her daughters to the SafePlace shelter. The police refused, however, to press charges against Jackson because they said Thomasina had "waited too long between the time of the assault and her call to them." They held the hours that she spent hiding in her daughter's bedroom against her. Yet again, the system had failed her in the most ludicrous and appalling way.

Her husband was eventually arrested and charged with the assault against Thomasina after the legal aide attorney assisting Thomasina with her divorce informed the courts there was an outstanding warrant against him on a day he was supposed to appear in court. He was never prosecuted for the assault because while waiting for the case to be docketed, he was arrested, charged, and found guilty of bank and mail fraud, for which he served prison time. When he was released from prison he was deported back to Nigeria, where he still resides.

Finally being accepted into the SafePlace shelter marked a turning point for Thomasina. Through counseling and support she began to put together the pieces of her life and to understand that she was not to blame for the abuse she had endured since early childhood. She began to learn she deserved only the best and to desire to live a truly empowered life. She also began to speak out about her prior victimization. When she spoke she realized that others looked at her and thought, "If she can find happiness, I can as well."

Thomasina, however, was still a single mom with four young children and no family or spousal support. Her travails were far from over. Sexual violence and domestic violence are both listed as causal factors in the backgrounds of many homeless women,[2] and Thomasina, despite having a master's degree, continued to teeter on the financial brink. Being accepted into shelter was an important first step, but it would take years for her to finally break free from the cycle of abuse and self-blame that dogged the first four decades of her life.

After two months in the shelter program, Thomasina and her daughters were accepted into the SafePlace transitional-housing program, which gave her eighteen months to stabilize her children and her life. She actively engaged in every aspect of the programming associated with transitional housing: attending individual and family counseling, taking part in life skills training, and working with her case manager to set and attain goals. She eventually landed a job with a local start-up company, a dot-com, as customer service manager, and moved with her girls into a rental house.

Unfortunately, Austin, a hub for the high-tech industry, was hit particularly hard in 2001 when the dot-com industry went bust. At first Thomasina held onto her job as others in the company were laid off, but eventually she, too, became unemployed. Again she collected unemployment benefits. Within weeks her landlord informed her that she would need to move because he had decided to sell the house. She had no money saved for a deposit and was within days of homelessness when we at Safe-Place received word of her plight. Thomasina didn't belong in the shelter and didn't qualify for transitional housing, but Angela Atwood, the director of transitional services, was determined to find a way to help her.

Several apartment communities in Austin worked with SafePlace to provide free or low-cost apartments on an occasional basis for families with special needs. Thomasina and her girls certainly fit the criteria. Within days we had secured an apartment for them, and once again Thomasina had the breathing room to rebuild her life. And once again — she did. This most amazing of women has earned all the happiness she now holds so dear — she has "kept the faith" through all of the bad times until she could create good times.

~

Each of these people — just a few of my personal heroes — could have been profoundly wounded for life. Instead, each has demonstrated remarkable survival skills. Why? There are no easy answers to that question, but I do see some similar patterns in their actions, values, and motivations. Each sought and found assistance to help them through difficult times: a supportive therapist, valued friends and family, and/or assistance from an agency such as SafePlace. In addition, each felt responsible for supporting and assisting others; they got outside of themselves. Donna, Thomasina, and Estrella each had young children to support and care for. Ed was truly healed when he found the daughter he had given up so many years before. Kimberly became a social worker and helped others to heal and grow.

Research on resiliency supports my own observations: Resilient people tend to be socially competent, especially as relates to the ability to elicit positive responses from others. They are flexible, possessing the ability to move between different cultures; are empathetic; are good communicators with the ability to create relationships; and have a sense of humor. And being of at least average intelligence helps with coping behavior. Smarter children have been found to be more resilient. In addition to being smart, Estrella, Donna, Kimberly, Ed, and Thomasina all have the gift of wisdom — a gift they each regularly use to help others.

Autonomy, or having a sense of one's own identity and an ability to act independently, to exert some control over one's destiny, is also associated with resiliency. The development of resistance, refusing to accept negative messages about oneself, and of detachment, or distancing oneself from dysfunction, also serve as a powerful protector of autonomy and a predictor of resiliency. When Thomasina ran away from home as a teenager she took control of her own destiny and refused to accept the negative messages she had received about her worth.

Lastly, research has shown that resiliency manifests in having a sense of purpose and a belief in a bright future.[3] Ed made helping SafePlace his purpose. Kimberly made helping others through social work her purpose. Thomasina, Donna, and Estrella all focused their attention on building better lives for their children. Almost all expressed a deeply held belief in God or a power greater than themselves. All are also naturally optimistic. Each of these individuals is blessed with a wonderful sense of humor and the ability and insight to look at their own actions, histories, and intentions — to decide to move forward with appreciation for the joy, beauty, and goodness they have found in everyday life.

7

the
batterer

*Thank you for helping me remember
who I am and that I have the right to
be happy, but also for not "punishing"
my ex-partner. He also needs help,
maybe more than me.*

— A survivor

I HAVE SPENT DECADES TRYING TO UNDERSTAND NOT ONLY MY decisions and behaviors but Jay's as well. Who are these men—yes, primarily men, and often good men in many aspects of their lives—who beat, rape, demean, and abuse women? Why do some men batter women? Many say it is because they drink or abuse other substances, or because they have a problem with anger management. Others say batterers have a psychological problem or trouble knowing how to communicate. Many say it is simply a learned behavior. I don't think the answer is so simple.

Jay's assaults on me increased when he was drunk, but even after he quit drinking his violent attacks and stalking continued. And he used communication as yet another tactic for assailing my self-esteem and ensuring my compliance with his demands. He could be an amazingly effective communicator; unfortunately, he often chose to use his communication skills as a means of violence. Yes, he certainly had anger management problems, but he didn't physically attack his work colleagues when they angered him; he waited to take his fury out on me. And yes, I believe he did in fact observe abuse as a child and had quite likely been the recipient of direct physical assaults. However, his brother, who had grown up in the same home, wasn't abusive to his wife. None of the above rationales can fully explain Jay's abusive behavior.

The primary reason why Jay, as well as other men who are abusive, attack women is because, quite simply, they can. When a man hits or yells at a woman, he is making a choice to do so. There are circumstances, like drinking, growing up with violence, and anger management problems, that make it more likely a man will abuse his partner, but there are no circumstances that can *make* a man attack his partner.

And battering works. It keeps a woman compliant and in the relationship, or from becoming involved in any other meaningful relationships. Women stay with abusive men because they know instinctually what research supports: The most dangerous time for a woman who is being battered is when she tries to leave.[1] A recent study of domestic violence–related deaths revealed that in 83 percent of the cases the victim was either separated or about to terminate the relationship.[2] In addition, verbal and emotional assaults may have so shattered a woman's self-esteem that she may doubt her value, judgment, and capabilities. When Jay called me "canyon cunt" he succeeded in holding me hostage. I was convinced that I was anatomically and sexually defective, and I was terrified of being with another man.

I remember a woman I encountered in my early years at Safehouse in Denver; she had been admitted to the hospital after a particularly brutal beating by her husband. When it came time for her to be released, she called a taxi to take her home. The cab driver who picked her up at the hospital had delivered many women to the front door of Safehouse over the years. Though most shelters are in confidential locations as a measure to keep women as safe as possible, most taxi drivers can tell you exactly where battered-women's shelters are located because they have taken so many women there—crying women, usually with young children in tow and a few belongings stuffed into plastic bags. They leave them at the locked front gate of a walled, secure facility often "hiding in plain sight" on a side street in an urban or suburban neighborhood. This particular cabbie, yet another anonymous hero, chose not to look away. He saw the woman's stitches, swelling, and bruises and said, "I'm sorry, ma'am, but I think you need to go someplace other than home, and I know just the place you should be." He drove her to Safehouse, rang the front doorbell, and said he hoped we would consider giving her shelter. We did.

She told us about the most recent assault, a beating she insisted she had deserved. She said, "I knew he didn't like tomatoes in his lettuce salad, so I should never have put them in." His ongoing attacks on her body and her self-esteem had so destroyed her personhood that she believed him when he said the beating was her fault because she'd put tomatoes on his salad! Her husband had usurped all power and control over her life. Sadly, she only stayed with us overnight, leaving the next day to return to him.

I have told this story countless times because it demonstrates one of the most basic facts about battering: It works. Battering is a very effective means of ensuring that a man can maintain power and control over another human being—most often the woman he claims to love.

Why, we have to ask, do some men want power and control? Why do they think it is their duty and their right to control the women in their lives?

Many men are not violent. In fact, a majority of men are not physically violent against women. And most men who are physically abusive to their partners are not monsters in other regards. Unfortunately, we live in a society that raises men to believe that aggression and violence are acceptable forms of self-expression. Young boys are encouraged to demonstrate strength and dominance rather than empathetic, caring, and nurturing attributes — characteristics that are devalued and seen as "feminine." How often do you hear a coach or a father deriding a little boy by saying, "You're throwing like a girl"? Even the governor of California, Arnold Schwarzenegger, has been widely quoted as mocking his state legislators, derisively calling them "girlie men." Such statements further reinforce the socialization that has taught boys that women are weak, unequal, and should be controlled, and that men are strong, powerful, and have the ability and the right to control others perceived as less powerful.

Sexism, that is, a belief in the inferiority of women, and a fear that a man's power may be diminished if the woman gains power, are at the core of violence against women. Brian Nichols, Public Policy Team Manager at Men Stopping Violence, based in Atlanta, Georgia, says, "Sexism is defined as gender prejudice plus power, the predisposition to experience women as inferior to men. Sexist norms and beliefs do not force any man to make the choice to be abusive, but they do provide the source from which such choices flow."

I will never understand why Jay was abusive to me. I know he displayed almost all of the characteristics that are identified with potential batterers. But these characteristics are indicative of the resulting behavior; they don't explain the "why."

Characteristics of a Batterer

Like most men who batter women, Jay was dependent on our relationship, emotionally even more than economically. Even after our divorce I continued to take responsibility for his actions, convinced that if I didn't help him he might end up homeless and dead, frozen on the side of a frigid winter Wyoming highway. He rationalized his use of violence and denied the severity of the abuse, both to me and to others, as do most men who batter. Abusive men also tend to believe in rigid sex roles, that men are superior and should be in charge of women. Although Jay was eager for me to work and generate income, he also held many sexist stereotypes that he'd picked up from his father, a career military man who was often stationed away from the family for months at a time. Jay would tell me lessons he'd learned from his father about women, such as, "Once you throw them down, roll them over, and stick it in, they're all the same."

Possessiveness and jealousy, sometimes to a pathological extent, are almost universal characteristics of men who batter. Jay told me that he was jealous because he "loved me so much." With time, I learned that jealousy has nothing to do with love; rather it is a sign of insecurity and possessiveness. Jay questioned me about whom I talked with, accused me of flirting, and was jealous of the time I spent with my family, friends, and children. He accused me of having affairs and other romantic interests, while in fact he was having affairs himself. Jay maintained that his constant surveillance and stalking were an effort to catch me in one of the dalliances he imagined I engaged in, even when we were no longer married.

Perpetrators of domestic violence will go to extreme lengths to isolate and control their partners. While I was with Jay I became alienated from almost all of my friends and family. At times, the isolation is taken to extremes. I have met women who were locked alone in their homes each day when their husbands went to work, left without access to phones or any other method of contacting the outside world, treated as the ultimate possession, mere objects to be cosseted and controlled at all costs.

Batterers are also described as having "Jekyll and Hyde" personalities that exhibit drastic contrasts. Much of the time they can be gentle and loving husbands and fathers. Jay could sometimes be the charming and devoted man I fell in love with and continued to love for several years. Many men consistently display their Dr. Jekyll side to the public, remaining smiling and friendly to those on the outside, only allowing Mr. Hyde to emerge at home. Luckily for me, the public occasionally witnessed Jay's Mr. Hyde personality, permitting others to believe him capable of the monstrous acts he committed at home.

I have already talked about Jay's alcohol abuse. Like many batterers, he displayed numerous addictive behaviors. In addition to alcohol abuse he smoked several packs of cigarettes a day. He started smoking marijuana when he woke in the morning and maintained a consistent high throughout each day, even after he had been through an alcohol-treatment program and ceased intake of all other types of drugs and alcohol.

Batterers often move too quickly in relationships. Jay pledged his undying love within days of our meeting. You'll remember that Thomasina, from the last chapter, was married within a few short months of meeting her first husband. Many survivors of domestic violence report they dated or knew their abuser for less than six months before they were living together. The abuser typically comes on like a whirlwind, claiming love at first sight and fulfilling a fantasy of fairytale romance. In textbook fashion Jay flattered me within weeks of our meeting with statements like, "I can't live without you."

An abusive man is usually hypersensitive, easily insulted, and claims hurt feelings when he is really feeling mad. A therapist will tell you that depression is anger turned inward. The opposite is also true. A batterer will take the slightest setback as a personal attack and will rant and rave about the injustice of things that have happened to him. Rarely did Jay accept responsibility for what happened in his life. He railed about losing his job because his boss was out to get him. He hit me because I bought sour cream, talked to another man, or questioned how he spent his day. I made him so mad he simply couldn't control himself. It was always someone else's fault. A lifelong pattern of avoiding the consequences of his behavior effectively limited his sense of personal responsibility for his destructiveness as well as suppressing any motivation to change. When he was thrown in jail for attacking my boss, his family made it my job to get him released immediately, in no way acknowledging my humiliation over the incident, nor recognizing that his actions might have warranted his spending some time in jail. Ensuring his success in life became my responsibility and, conversely, I also became responsible for all of his failures.

Men who batter will often initiate or agree to attend counseling in order to keep their partner in the relationship, but rarely, at least initially, in order to change themselves. They will often end the counseling once their partner returns to the relationship, a new relationship is established, or the mandate from a criminal-justice agency has been lifted. But without intensive counseling directed at the batterer's behavior, the violence is likely to continue.

The strongest indicator that a man will batter his wife is if he has hit women previously, breaks or strikes objects, threatens violence, and/or uses any force during an argument. A woman may hear from relatives or ex-partners that the man is abusive, but she wants to believe that it will be different this time. He will tell her, "She made me do it. It won't be like that with you. You're different" — thus putting the responsibility for his actions back on his partner.

The man may also make violent threats — "I'll kill you," "I'll cut your head off and bury it in the backyard," "I'll take your children and you will never see them again" — and then say, "Everybody talks like that." *They don't.* And the validity of these threats should never be underestimated. Studies have shown that previous threats to kill the partner are a significant predictor of lethality in a relationship.

Breaking or striking objects is often used as a punishment and as a physical threat. Jay regularly destroyed my possessions and broke things around me as a way of terrorizing me into submission. Holding a woman down, physically restraining her from leaving the room, pushing, shoving, and any physical force during an argument should be a flashing red warning light. As with my marriage, throwing things at the wall often escalates to throwing things at the woman, and worse.

The man will often refuse to seek help for his behaviors unless the woman agrees to go with him, a tactic that again suggests the woman shares responsibility for her partner's violence, all too often reinforced by the professional counseling community. Many couples will end up seeking couples counseling or mediation, an intervention that most domestic-violence advocates will strongly advise against as the initial or primary intervention for battering, stating that it may not be safe to talk about feelings in front of someone who could hurt you later and blame his behavior on what you say. However, a basic philosophy of the battered-women's movement is that a woman should be allowed to make her own decisions about her life, even if the advocate does not agree. I believe it is our responsibility as advocates to make every effort to listen to the woman and be responsive to her needs and wishes—which may, at some point, mean couples counseling in an environment as structured and as safe as possible, which may necessitate having an advocate present and/or a counselor specifically trained in and knowledgeable about the dynamics of battering.

Jay's abusive behavior, like the behavior of batterers from around the world, was reinforced by institutions and cultural mores that promote sexist messages about women, validating an abusive man's beliefs that he has the right and authority to control his wife. Two traditions that are seldom questioned but are firmly rooted in men's ownership of women is that of the father giving away the bride and of the bride taking her husband's name. When I first married Jay I never questioned that I would take his last name as my own. However, I began to question it when people started regularly referring to me as Mrs. Jay Smith. I felt as though I was suddenly perceived as an addendum to my husband—as though my personhood had disappeared. When I tried to explain my feelings to Jay and the fact that I didn't want to be called Mrs. Jay Smith, but rather to retain my own independent and unique identity, he reacted as though I were denouncing our marriage and his rights. Another man, including my current husband, might have said, "I understand your concerns and I will work with you to ensure that you don't become an afterthought or addendum to me." Jay's reaction was to rein me in tighter by whatever means he could. I have many good friends who have thoughtfully chosen to take their husband's last names because it is easier, particularly when there are young children involved. I sometimes question the wisdom of my own choice to maintain my last name when I married my current husband, Bill McLellan. Listening to our home answering machine you hear such a long list of last names that we have had people think they have reached a law firm in error!

Institutions such as churches, courts, schools, and hospitals have often unwittingly colluded with batterers to reinforce the notions of men's superiority and women's inferiority. Many churches still don't consider women worthy of leadership roles, and some police officers still ask battered women, "What did you do to make him hit you?"

I once met a woman who quit attending her long-time church to show support for a friend who was married to a deacon, a pious and respected member of the congregation who also abused his wife regularly. The woman told me of seeing the husband hit his wife one day at church as they stood in a side room, believing they were alone and his actions wouldn't be observed. The woman I was talking to took the information to the lead pastor of the church, asking that someone intervene to assist the wife. She was told that it wasn't church business. Later, after yet another abusive incident, the husband said to his wife, "Come over here, baby. Let's kiss and make up." When she approached him, *the husband bit off her bottom lip.* Since she required emergency care and the criminal-justice system became involved, the husband's assaults against his wife were no longer a well-kept secret. The wife, now horribly disfigured, returned to her church home, hoping for solace and emotional support. Instead, she was asked by the church leadership to please quit attending services because it was too embarrassing to her husband for everyone to see her mutilated face.

At the same time, over the last few decades many institutions have begun to step up and institute structural and behavioral changes to support victims and hold perpetrators accountable. Almost all of these changes have come about because of the work of victim rights groups and the battered-women's and feminist movements. In 1983 Jay's right of ownership was reinforced by the police officer who failed to write a report because I was Jay's former wife. But in the late 1990s, when stopped by a police officer as I sped too fast across northwestern Oklahoma on the way to my brother's funeral in Dodge City, Kansas, I was pleasantly surprised when the highway patrolman asked me to please step to the back of the car, away from my second husband, who was sitting beside me in the front seat. He'd noted that I had a black eye, so he separated me from my husband to ask if I needed assistance. From this incident I learned what a difference a decade had made. I wish I knew the officer's name so I could acknowledge him now. (And, yes, different husband, different state, different life, and I had a black eye. I learned the hard way that sometimes when a woman tells you she ran into a door — she might have really run into a door. While helping with my brother during his final days, I had taken his dog out for a walk. The eager pup, once leashed, had literally leapt out the door, pulling me face first into the open door-jamb.)

Batterer's-Intervention Programs

In addition to institutional responses to domestic violence, a plethora of batterer's programs have been established in the last couple of decades. Often these programs have been initiated at the behest of criminal-justice systems that, required to hold batterers accountable and overwhelmed by the sheer volume of cases, are desperate for options other than over-crowded jails and prisons. In addition, the courts recognize that jailing a perpetrator may increase the hardship on the family by taking away its only viable means of support.

I am often asked, "Do batterer's-treatment programs work?" I have no easy answer. My personal observation is that these programs can and do work to help keep women safe if a basic tenet of the program is about holding their partners accountable for their actions. I have seen men change their abusive behaviors, though often it is too late for the rela-tionship that brought them into the treatment program. The programs are most effective when the man voluntarily enters the program, is com-mitted to changing, and fully participates. If a man isn't truly committed to being accountable for his behavior and to stop being controlling, he is unlikely to change his behavior, with or without a batterer's program.

Any batterer's program should prioritize the safety of the victim/ survivor first, thus requiring some limitations on client confidentiality, which is a significant break from traditional therapy practice. The perpetrator should sign a release of information to the victim/survivor permitting staff to advise her of her partner's enrollment, attendance, any ongoing threats of violence, discharge, and program completion. The program should maintain the victim's confidentiality, never disclosing information about her without her permission to do so. A release should also be given to the appropriate court worker when the court has mandated participation.

Again, in a significant break from traditional therapy practice, the batterer should be directly confronted about his abusive behaviors and not allowed to minimize or make excuses. If the batterer says he "didn't really hit her that hard," the facilitator may confront him with medical reports or photos, effectively disputing his account of events.

A batterer's program should be both process-driven and education-driven. The participant must first learn to recognize abuse before he can begin to unlearn his battering behaviors. The program should provide information that helps men understand the dynamics of domestic violence within the context of cultural learning and male socialization. All beliefs or attitudes employed to justify the use of violence in intimate relationships, especially the perceived right to dominate or control women, should be challenged. Programs that address only his anger, communication skills, or stress do not get to the root of the problem. Participants must learn how their violence affects their female partners and their relationships, its impact on children, and its effect on other family members witnessing the violence. The program should enable participants to acknowledge their violent behavior, take responsibility for it, and initiate positive change within their personal relationships.

A man who is sincerely committed to change will need to be trained on egalitarian, respectful strategies for decision-making, communication, and conflict resolution. He will need to learn how to have an intimate emotional relationship and to identify and express feelings respectfully. He should learn discussion versus argument, honesty versus deception, how to build bridges rather than walls, and to "do unto others as they would like to be done to," rather than "do unto others before they do unto me." The program should emphasize that lasting behavioral change is the measure of successful completion of the program, not simply finishing a certain number of sessions.[3]

Not all batterers are alike, and not all types of batterers are equally likely to respond to treatment programs. Furthermore, not all batterer's programs are held to the same standards, and, in a field desperate for solutions and with potential for income generation from fees and taxpayer dollars, many men are diverted into treatment programs that may not be effective. In fact, at times they may prove harmful.

Institutional and Treatment Approaches to Battering

Two professors at the University of Washington, Dr. John Gottman and Dr. Neil Jacobson, conducted a ten-year study of two hundred couples, sixty of which were studied intensively. They identified two different categories of abusive men, and how the distinction can make a difference in the severity of the harm they inflict, the ability of women to escape a relationship, the risks the women face if they do leave, and the potential for successful intervention in the batterer's behavior. "O. J. Simpson," they reported, "is a classic pit bull, a man who mostly confines his monstrous behavior to the woman he professes to love, acting out of emotional dependence and a fear of abandonment. Pit bulls are the stalkers, the jealous husbands and boyfriends who are charming to everyone except their wives and girlfriends. Cobras, on the other hand, are often cold and calculating sociopaths. Cobras are the ones who kill the cat as a warning to wives that if they fail to toe the mark, this could happen to them." Dr. Jacobson says the best place for cobras is prison. However, an abused wife is often most in danger from a "pit bull" rather than a "cobra." The sociopathic "cobra" may not have the emotional dependence on his partner and will simply move on to another, easier victim if his partner is successful in getting away from him.

I have spent considerable time trying to decide which of these two categories Jay fit into, and I believe he would have been classified by Gottman and Jacobson as a "pit bull." He wasn't consistently charming to everyone but me, but his abusive behavior was almost totally based on maintaining his control over me. He could also be genuinely distressed over his behaviors, unlike the "cobra," a sociopath unable to feel remorse.

Dr. Jacobson also says, "If the laws were different and enforced differently, battered women would be much safer. If wife-beating was an automatic felony and the perpetrators had a mandatory jail sentence, women would have a chance to experience life without an abusive man and to formulate a safety plan to escape from the relationship." Dr. Daniel Saunders, at the University of Michigan School of Social Work, has said, "The evidence thus far indicates that a combination of arrest, prosecution, fines, and counseling works better than any one approach alone."[4] However, our criminal-justice systems are already overloaded, and the system would collapse from the sheer weight of the numbers if all wife-beaters were prosecuted as felons.

In Chicago's Cook County court system, more than nineteen thousand domestic abuse cases are handled each year. In 1997 the state's attorney launched a program to identify and actively pursue the most serious misdemeanor domestic-violence cases; prosecutors say convictions in those cases soared to as high as 73 percent. But even so, resources for the program are so limited that a federally funded review found that the program was pursuing only thirty of ninety offenders identified each week as being at high risk of committing murder.[5] Unfortunately, sometimes batterers who have not been prosecuted by the special program have gone on to murder the women they were abusing. The situation in Cook County isn't unusual; in almost every jurisdiction across the country the criminal-justice system is unable to deal with the sheer number of similar cases and has instead developed ineffective means of trying to move people through the system. That becomes the primary goal rather than ensuring safety for women and families.

I used to carry a Polaroid snapshot of a battered woman in my wallet. I regularly pulled it out to dramatically demonstrate the types of domestic violence that were being prosecuted as misdemeanors — that is, at the same level as urinating in public. The woman in the photograph had a broken nose, two black eyes, and a split lip, and her neck was completely encircled by dark bruises. Choking a victim has been correlated with potential lethality in a relationship. A similar assault committed by a stranger or against almost anyone other than the man's wife would have certainly resulted in a more serious charge. The severity of the bruising around her neck surely indicated attempted murder. However, a prison sentence would have deprived the family of its primary breadwinner and denied the batterer the opportunity to benefit from a batterer's program. There are no easy answers — in saving a woman's life we may also be sentencing a family to a life of destitution.

A young man who became involved with SafePlace through Expect Respect, a school-based program designed to teach youth about healthy relationships, was the first man ever hired by SafePlace to work in the shelter. He was referred to the agency because of concerns about domestic violence in his dating relationship. He actively participated in the group, became a peer leader, volunteered, and was eventually hired to work in the children's services component of the shelter program. He considers working with men to end domestic violence and sexual assault his life's work. Yes, a motivated man can unlearn controlling and abusive behaviors and become a good husband, teacher, and role model.

Despite an accumulation of studies evaluating programs for offenders, firm conclusions cannot be made yet about the effectiveness of intervention,[6] but, anecdotally, I have seen men learn to be different. My suggestion to anyone genuinely seeking assistance with battering behaviors would be to call the National Domestic Violence Hotline at (800) 799-SAFE (7233) or (800) 787-3224 (TTY) and ask for referrals in your local area.

Jay may have successfully made that transition. I don't know. Despite our sons and shared history, I have never delved into the life he built following our divorce. I do know that he had the desire to live differently. And I have to believe that all of us have the ability to learn and grow and change.

the youngest survivors: children and domestic violence

I feel sad when my mom and my dad fight. He hit my mom with the electric fan.

— A child talking about his parents

MY SONS' MEMORIES HAVE FADED—THEY NO LONGER CARRY any recollections of the crazy, scary times of their early childhoods. But I will always worry that those years left indelible imprints on their psyches. I once overheard five-year-old Cody, always outgoing and articulate, telling a neighbor that his "daddy used to beat up my mommy." He also told his little brother Brandon about huddling with him under the stairs, trying to hide him from his daddy "when he was mad." Even if they no longer retain the conscious memories, those were my sons' formative years.

I recognize that I am not able to honestly assess the impact of the abuse on my sons. When I read the literature about infants and preschool-age children who are living in homes with domestic violence, my immediate reaction is one of denial. This chapter was almost impossible for me to research and write.

Psychosocial Characteristics of Children
Living in Homes with Domestic Violence

"The physical and psychological needs of infants are unmet or only inconsistently addressed."[1] This is just one of the impacts of domestic violence on families that were noted by the children's counseling staff at SafePlace. But certainly, I try to convince myself, it was not the case with my children; I loved my babies and did everything in my power to make sure they were cared for.

Then I recall the times when I was sick from a stress-induced migraine and unable to get out of bed or adequately attend to my children's needs. I remember putting the boys into bed with me, giving them bottles to comfort them, and turning on a children's cartoon on the bedroom television at the lowest possible volume. I would burrow my head under a pillow and try to ignore every aspect of a world that seemed to be tearing my head apart from the inside out. Then there was the time that I broke my ankle and would have gladly welcomed Count Dracula into my home if only he would help me with my infant and toddler sons.

SafePlace materials also state, "The infant may not be able to form a strong trust with the parent and often has higher incidences of illness,

150

irritability, and sleep difficulties."[2] I jokingly say, "Cody has never slept through the night; he just got old enough that I didn't have to get up with him anymore." I remember a Wyoming winter night when I awakened to the sound of my three-year-old son's cries. Pulling myself out of my warm cocoon of a bed I went to see what was wrong and found that Cody had awakened in the night and wandered into the attached but unheated garage. Had I not wakened to his crying, he could have easily frozen to death in the sub-zero cold. Cody's sleep was always erratic and troubled, a fact I never wanted to attribute to the violence he saw in his home. And I have already written about the crippling asthma that plagued Brandon's infancy despite what I thought were my best efforts to protect him from triggers and to religiously maintain his medication schedule. When I left Laramie, Brandon's asthma dramatically improved. Did he "grow out of it," as I have often said, or was it his improved living environment once I finally fled his father?

Advocates point out that in homes with domestic violence, "Toddlers often lack consistent discipline and have problems with boundaries and limit setting, they may not show a healthy level of independence, and they may rely on acting out to express [their] feelings."[3] This was certainly my experience with Cody as a toddler and one of the factors that influenced my decision to leave my home, my job, my friends, and my state in order to protect myself and my children. Cody acted out in the only ways available to a two- or three-year-old child.

He was also extremely attuned to my emotions and fears. I particularly remember the day I drove home after yet another difficult encounter with Jay. I was trying to consider the options available to me and thinking that perhaps I could move to Wichita, Kansas. Wichita was located relatively close to my parents, so they might be able to provide some assistance with the boys, and it was large enough that I could probably find a job. At that moment, three-year-old Cody, sitting in his car seat behind me, said, "Mom, why don't we move to Wichita so we can be close to Grandma and Grandpa?" Could my son read my mind? Had I inadvertently said something that signaled my thoughts? I don't know—but I do know that my little boy felt responsible for protecting and taking care of his mother. This wasn't the way things were supposed to be.

Even when domestic violence doesn't result in direct physical injury to a child, it can interfere with both a mother's and a father's parenting to such a degree that the child may be neglected. Though many parents believe that they hide the violence from their children, children living in these homes report differently. Research conducted during the 1980s suggests that between 80 and 90 percent of children are aware of the battering.[4] Even if they don't see a beating, they hear the screams and see the bruises, broken bones, and abrasions sustained by their mothers. During the past decade, juvenile and family courts have struggled to understand the significance of child exposure when making decisions concerning custody and visitation. All parties involved are recognizing the need for better methods to assess such exposure.

I have tried to convince myself that my sons didn't suffer any permanent psychological harm from the chaos they lived through in their early years, but I must also admit that, no, I wasn't always the mother I hoped to be and the mother that my sons needed and deserved.

Historically, little research has been dedicated to studying the traumatic impact of domestic violence on children and the implications of that trauma on a child's later life. Additionally, any research has been complicated by the difficulty in differentiating the effects of living in a violent home from all of the other indicators that are often present in abusive families. Children living in poverty are often forced to move repeatedly and change schools repeatedly; they feel isolated and live in fear from street gangs and other dangers that may lurk outside their doors. The living conditions associated with economic insecurity and poverty, for the most part, closely mirror the conditions associated with living in a violent home. The major difference, of course, is the haven of a loving parental relationship, being safe from the fear of threats from within the supposed refuge of home.

Studies of children exposed to the violence of war provide some insights into the probable impact on children living with parental violence. These studies have consistently shown that separation from family and the destruction of important early relationships is one of the most potentially damaging consequences of war for children. But the children in war zones who are cared for by their own parents or familiar adults have been found to suffer far fewer negative effects.[5] These studies demonstrate the importance of a parent in providing a stable and consistent role in a child's life, a role that may be compromised if the parent is severely traumatized from domestic violence. Even if a child has not witnessed or been the direct recipient of abuse, he or she will likely feel the impact of the traumatized and battered parent.

The Long-Term Impact of Domestic Violence on Children

Some studies have produced troubling results that indicate ongoing effects even after the home environment has improved. In a 2005 study, researchers looked at what impact interpersonal violence had on people as children by observing their mental-health outcomes in adulthood. The researchers measured current depression and lifetime suicide attempts, intimate-partner violence, violence against children, and alcohol dependence. They asked participants about childhood adversities, such as parental separation, divorce, parental death or imprisonment, alcoholism, and physical and/or sexual abuse, and about social stressors, including poor parental health, housing problems, prolonged parental unemployment, and financial troubles. Among the group of people interviewed, 16 percent said they had witnessed interparental violence before the age of eighteen, and this was far more common in certain situations. For example, it was up to eight times more likely in cases where parents had been alcoholics. Witnessing violence was also more common in families with financial problems, serious parental diseases, housing problems, or unemployment.

After adjusting for family- and social-level stressors, the researchers found that people who had witnessed violence between their parents had a 40 percent higher risk of depression, were 3 times more likely to be involved in violence in an intimate or marital relationship, were almost

5 times more likely to mistreat their own child, and were 1.75 times more likely to have dependence on alcohol.[6]

In a 2008 study conducted by the University of Rochester, the University of Minnesota, and the University of Notre Dame, researchers tried to determine whether children who showed specific behavior patterns of reacting to conflict also had changes in levels of cortisol, a hormone associated with stress. The researchers simulated telephone arguments between the children's parents and then measured the children's distress, hostility, and level of involvement in the arguments. They also received reports from the mothers about how their children responded when parents fought at home. Cortisol was measured by taking saliva samples from the children both before and after the simulated conflicts. Children who were very distressed by the conflicts had higher levels of cortisol in response to their parent's fighting. Children who were both very distressed and very involved in parental fighting had especially high levels of cortisol.

According to the leader of the study, Patrick T. Davies, professor of psychology at the University of Rochester, "Our results indicate that children who are distressed by conflict between their parents show greater biological sensitivity to conflict in the form of higher levels of the stress hormone, cortisol. Because higher levels of cortisol have been linked to a wide range of mental- and physical-health difficulties, high levels of cortisol may help explain why children who experience high levels of distress when their parents argue are more likely to experience later health problems."[7]

Does this research mean that children raised in violent homes are inevitably doomed to becoming dysfunctional adults: suicidal, depressed, alcoholic, and abusive? Will they always live on the edge, with increased levels of cortisol keeping them in a constant state of "fight or flight"? My oldest son, Cody, is a rock climber, scaling the sides of cliffs, clinging with toes and fingertips to holds that are invisible to the untrained eye — often little more than tiny fissures in the rock or millimeter-wide protuberances. His proclivity for rock climbing, a daring sport by almost anyone's standards, might be attributed to the high cortisol levels he developed as a little boy, hiding with his brother under the stairs. I also remember the baby boy who was climbing out of his crib and scaling the kitchen cabinets even before he could walk.

A 1999 study at the University of Michigan leaves me with more hope that the dysfunctional state of affairs in our home didn't permanently scar my young sons. The study indicated that reducing the frequency of violent acts children are subjected to can relieve the odds of a youngster's having painful, intrusive, post-traumatic stress symptoms. Those with intrusive symptoms witnessed about seventeen "severe" violent acts (punching, beating up, weapon use) and twenty-three "mild" ones (slapping and shoving). Children without intrusive symptoms saw about one severe act and four mildly violent ones. Sandra Graham-Bermann, a psychologist at the University of Michigan, Ann Arbor, states, "For some, it's not post-traumatic stress. It's more like chronic stress because violence is so frequent."[8]

Battered Women as Perpetrators of Child Abuse

My primary blame lies in my inaction, but children whose mothers are abused sometimes suffer at the hands of their mothers as well. Mothers are more likely to neglect or abuse their children while they are in an abusive relationship. One study found that women were eight times more likely to hurt their children while they themselves were being battered than after they left the abusive relationship.[9] Sometimes a mother may hurt her children as a means of trying to protect herself and them in the face of threats like, "If you don't keep those kids quiet I'm going to hurt them and you." Other seemingly neglectful behaviors on the part of the mother may be a direct result of battering. I know of mothers being prevented from taking their children to school because school personnel might report the child's injuries. Thus, the mother becomes complicit in the abuse against the child. The abused woman may also be overwhelmed by the injuries and stress of her own abuse, compromising her abilities to parent effectively.

Battered women who also abuse their children for whatever reason are particularly reluctant to ask for help. They are afraid, deservedly so, that in seeking assistance they may lose custody of their children. I know a woman who is in a very abusive marriage and, after a vicious verbal assault by both her husband and his mother, bit her hysterical toddler. Yes, this intelligent and accomplished woman bit her daughter. I don't pretend to understand the impulse that drove her to such an action, but I do know that it haunted her for years. Her mother-in-law promptly, and correctly, called the police to report child abuse, and an extensive investigation ensued. The investigation didn't result in any action, but the mother was now on the record as the perpetrator of an assault against her child. In the years ahead, whenever she considered trying to escape the battering, she was reminded that she would never get custody of their children because she had been investigated for child abuse. The woman lives with her husband to this day, convinced that leaving him will result in her losing her children. I would suggest that her best option might be to proactively engage in parenting classes and demonstrate her capability as a parent, showing decision-makers that she will be an effective parent in the future and deserves to maintain custody of her children.

Children as Perpetrators

My sons were no longer being exposed to domestic violence by the time they reached school age. But children of all ages are deeply affected by domestic abuse, and school-age children who witness violence may exhibit violence toward their peers. Adolescents, in particular, who have grown up in violent homes are at risk for re-creating the abusive relationships they have seen.[10]

Children who are bullies, and those who have been bullied, have also been identified as potential perpetrators of violence. Like battered women, children who have been bullied may strike back or defend themselves with a weapon, thus inflicting greater harm.

Supporting Children

One of the most important things we can do in support of children living in homes with domestic violence is to help them learn how to protect themselves. Children should not be burdened with the responsibilities of managing or predicting their parents' behavior, but neither should they be left with no means or strategies for coping with situations in which they don't feel safe. As discussed earlier, even when you think they don't know, children are almost always aware of domestic violence in the home and of the attendant tension and fear.

Talk with children about the times they feel scared and what they think they might be able to do to help them feel better. Openly discussing the child's anxieties while simultaneously trying not to cause additional alarm is a tricky balance. Tell the child it isn't their fault and they shouldn't feel responsible for their father's anger, but there are some things they might do to help themselves feel safer: Run out of the home when the incident starts, stay out of the room where there is fighting, stay out of the kitchen and garage where it is easier to get hurt, and stay out of small rooms like a bathroom or closet where they could be trapped. Talk with the child to help determine in advance a safe place where the child might be able to go, like a neighbor's or friend's house, or a prearranged code word to use with friends or relatives so they can use the phone to call for help without the abuser knowing what they are doing. Children should also be taught how to call 911. Reinforce the idea that the abuse is not their fault and that it is okay to love both parents even if one is hurting the other, but that it is never okay for one parent to hurt the other, the child, or someone else. Unfortunately, the only way to truly relieve the child of the fear and burden of abuse is to end or escape the abuse.

Child Custody and Domestic Violence

After a woman leaves a batterer, it has been tragically common for family courts to require women to send their children on unsupervised visits with their abusive fathers, even in cases where there is an extensive and well-documented history of domestic violence, often including threats to use the children to manipulate or control the woman. It is impossible to convey the level of despair expressed by one woman whose abusive former husband had taken the children for court-approved visitation, strapped them into their car seats in his car, and murdered them by pumping carbon monoxide into a cracked window from a hose attached to the car's exhaust. The ex-husband, also dead, in the front seat, left a note addressed to his wife: "If I can't have them, no one will." I knew this woman. I saw her anguish. I also saw her become an advocate for other battered women and children. She led the fight to educate the courts to save the lives of other children.

In the past decade, family courts have seen enormous reform. All states must now consider domestic violence in custody and visitation decisions, but only about half of them make it the primary consideration. Legal innovations include protections for survivors who need to relocate due to safety concerns, and exemptions from mandated mediation. However, many states still have "friendly parent" statutes that do not recognize battered women's reluctance to co-parent. Domestic-violence training materials and guidelines are increasingly available for judges, court managers, custody evaluators, and parenting coordinators, but this training should be mandated for all family court and evaluation personnel. Accessible and affordable supervised visitation centers should also be made available.

Jay didn't fight me when I requested that visitation with our sons be supervised. His willingness to comply enabled my sons to have a relationship with their father without the stress and fear always present when their father and I interacted. It also allowed me to feel a measure of comfort in their safety and well-being. Not all children are so lucky. Despite the measures cited above, children continue to be compelled to spend unsupervised visitations with controlling and abusive fathers. When this happens, again give the children a chance to talk about their fears and their ideas about keeping themselves safe. Ask them to think through the setup at their father's home and about how to get to a phone and to a safe place. Make sure the children know their home phone number by heart and how to call for help. Children need to know that they should always make their own safety their top priority. If the father pumps the child for information about the mom, let them know that they can tell him what he is asking about—but that they should let the mom know what they have said so she can prepare for his reaction to a new boyfriend or a job outside the home. A particularly difficult issue, and one I have encountered, is protecting your children from getting into a car with their father when he is intoxicated or high. I have refused to allow my sons to leave with their father because I didn't trust him behind the wheel, sparking an episode of uncontrolled rage targeted at me. But what if the mother is not there to monitor the situation and the children are too young to speak for themselves? There are no easy answers. Most important, remind the child that they are in no way to blame for their parents' actions.

If a parent is involved in court litigation with an ex-partner over custody or visitation, the fact that the mother has talked with the children about safety planning can be used against her. The father may claim that she has been instilling fear into the children and trying to alienate them from him. In these instances it is best to arrange with a professional to talk with the child about safety planning, rather than doing it oneself. This can usually be coordinated with a therapist or through a local battered-women's program.

Unfortunately, I have seen women use allegations of abuse as a means of undermining a father's relationship with his child, or of trying to gain the upper hand in a divorce proceeding. Women who use these tactics undermine the safety of many other women and children by providing fodder for militant father's rights groups and opening the door to the questioning of all battered women fighting for the safety of their children. The relatively rare instances of women making up these allegations should never be used as an excuse for suspecting all women and putting children in danger.

Children and Teens: Learning New Behaviors

Children of all ages who are living in homes with domestic violence learn to keep secrets, learn to use aggression and manipulation to get what they want, and learn that violence is a normal and acceptable part of life. School-age children and teens may assign gender roles as witnessed in their household: the male as aggressive, violent, and powerful, the female as weak, submissive, and a victim. They may show signs of intolerance of differences in others, may align themselves with the parent who has the power, and may begin to repeat the cycle of abuse in their own dating relationships.

Violence-prevention programs targeting teen-dating relationships are generally designed to work with teens living in homes with domestic violence, as well as with teens engaged in abusive-dating relationships. They differ from other violence-prevention programs in that they insert an important gender-based perspective into the discussions surrounding expectations and relationships for today's teens—expectations that I think are increasingly more intense and pervasive but that have been present to some extent for a very long time.

While in high school I went "riding around" and drinking beer with several friends in a football player's old Scout four-wheel drive. There were three girls and four boys; most of us were friends and hung out together often. But in a very odd twist, probably associated with the beer, couples started pairing off and, in the lingo of my day, "making out," which at that time meant heavy necking. I remember sitting huddled against the front door feeling a bit appalled for my friends and wondering what was going on. When we stopped for a pit stop at a gas station and I ran into the restroom with one of my girlfriends, she said to me, "Kelly, they bought us beer and are driving us around. We owe it to them to make out with them." I perceived the friend who made this comment as being much more popular and together than I, and yet she was saying something that made no sense to me at all. I quickly questioned my beliefs and values. Was I wrong to think that no quid pro quo was implied through a night spent together partying? When we returned to the car my friend paired off with another of the boys and I stayed huddled in my corner of the front seat. These boys were my friends and I can very honestly say that I never for a moment feared that any one of them would force himself on me—but what is wrong when a young girl thinks that buying her a beer, a nice dinner, or an evening out requires the gift of her physical affections? And how many young men think that is the way the game is played and that when the girl doesn't put out it is his right to take his due by any means available?

These complicated rules of relationships and courtships have become even more difficult and complex for young people today, particularly with the advent of social media, and almost every parent struggles with how to protect their teens and help them build the judgment and skills to protect themselves. There are certainly no magical words or potions that will protect our children from the misogynistic and violent messages that abound in today's world. However, the National Teen Dating Abuse Hotline ([866] 331-9474 or TTY [866] 331-8453) says that parents and adult mentors can make a difference. They recommend that adults first analyze their own dating values before speaking with their teens. Think about how you expect men and women to act in a relationship and whether you are modeling that behavior. How should decisions be made and disagreements handled? Needless to say, if a parent is in an abusive and disrespectful relationship, it is doubtful their word will carry much weight with their offspring.

Children and teens learn by observing those around them, especially their parents. At the core of every violence-prevention program, both intimate partner and otherwise, is respect for yourself, your partner, and other people.

9

shelters

The first time I came to the shelter I was so filled with shame that I could not look up or accept help, I had to go home.

The second time I came to the shelter I was so angry that I was the one who had to leave my home that I was like a raging elephant. My anger fell on everyone around me, I could not hear advice or accept help.

The third time I came to the shelter, I was open to accepting the help that was offered.

— A SafePlace shelter client

I WAS LUCKY. WHEN I MADE A CALL REQUESTING EMERGENCY shelter from a pay phone outside a convenience store, a real person answered the phone, told me space was available, and encouraged me to come right over. Thomasina, whose story appears in Chapter 6, had a more typical experience. Despite her situation being every bit as serious as mine, when she first called SafePlace she was told the shelter was full and her name could only be put on a waiting list.

You are probably wondering how a crisis program can operate with a waiting list. The very nature of "crisis" should make the idea of a waiting list unthinkable. But in Texas in 2006 over 22 percent of requests for shelter were turned away or placed on a waiting list because the shelter called was already full.[1] And in my experience, Texas has a more comprehensive network of battered-women's programs than most states. If it is that bad in Texas, how much worse must it be elsewhere?

Austin's SafePlace, like every shelter in the United States, has always struggled to ensure that no one is ever turned away or placed on a waiting list without initial efforts to assess immediate danger, provide safety planning, and discuss options for alternative shelter. However, assessing immediate danger can be a very inexact and dangerous process. I used to hold my breath every time I heard of a domestic homicide in Central Texas, hoping against hope I wouldn't discover that the victim had attempted to get into our shelter and been turned away because the shelter was full. To my knowledge, this has not yet happened.

Since the first battered-women's shelter opened its doors, women have lined up seeking protection for themselves and their children. Most often, the requests for shelter far outpace the space and resources available, necessitating some kind of process for delineating admission criteria, how long a woman can stay, and the actions she must take while in the shelter.

Why a Battered-Women's Shelter?

Shelter is about survival first, and all shelter programs necessarily place a large emphasis on safety and crisis management. When it comes to decisions about admission, I believe the number-one criterion for every battered-women's shelter should always be safety: Is this woman and/or her children in immediate danger, is alternative safe shelter available, can the program keep her and her children safe, will her admission put other shelter residents and/or staff at undue risk? If she cannot be kept safe in our facility, might she be housed safely elsewhere?

For the most part, each shelter operates as a private, nonprofit corporation, governed by a local independent board of directors, and with its own policies and procedures, yet the programs also operate as a network, maintaining a loose web of services and attempting to create safe places for battered women and their children across the country. When it was apparent that Estrella, the woman who was shot five times as she tried to escape her husband, could not be kept safe in Dallas, her home community, she was transferred to SafePlace in Austin in hopes that her husband wouldn't be able to find her there. Such transfers happen every day across communities, states, and the nation.

Many years ago I hid a woman's car, a distinctive make and model, in my home garage. She and her three children had been moved multiple times between shelters and across several states in an attempt to thwart the efforts of her drug-dealer husband to locate them and make good on his promise to their son to "cut off your mother's head and bury it in the backyard if she ever tries to get away." She had given up all contact with her family and friends, fled to a city she had never visited and where she knew no one, dyed her hair and that of her children, changed all of their names, and disappeared into a totally new and different world. Her preadolescent children lived in fear that their father would discover their new names and where they had run to—a fact that dramatically underscored the validity of her fears. Her situation was so dangerous that police officers even advised us that they probably could not keep her safe. And contrary to portrayals in the popular media, battered-women's shelters don't generally have the capacity and ability to secretly and legally change women's identities. Almost all official avenues for changing an identity leave a record somewhere that a determined man with sufficient resources can use to track down his spouse.

Not every case is so dramatic, but these are the stories that make the news and about which TV movies are made, resulting in many women not calling a shelter because they think their situation isn't severe enough. But no one should ever hesitate to call because they "aren't abused badly enough." The hotline can provide referrals to other agencies, assist with safety planning, and help to assess the level of danger.

At other times I have been amazed that a woman hasn't been advised that she should enter a shelter to try to keep herself, her family, and her friends safe. Again, I was lucky that someone told me it wouldn't be safe for me, or for my friends, if I went once again to their house and that I really needed to seek emergency shelter.

I remember when a woman from Central Texas was tracked to her sister's apartment, where she was shot by her husband and left permanently brain damaged. He then kidnapped their baby daughter and fled with her to another state. He was eventually tracked down and died in a shoot-out with the police. His daughter was in the car with him; thankfully, she was spared. All of this occurred after the husband had broken into his in-laws' home and killed his mother-in-law while searching for his wife and child. The police never advised the young wife to go to a shelter. I later became friends with the wife's father, a quiet, melancholy man who was dealing with the violent loss of his wife while caring for his adult daughter, disabled from the attack, and also raising his granddaughter. He regularly spoke out to other young women and to families, encouraging them to recognize the urgency of abusive marriages and to seek the support of domestic-violence programs.

Making the Call for Help

Every admission to the SafePlace shelter, as with most shelters, is preceded by a phone call. The woman personally calls the hotline asking for assistance and often for admission. She may be making the call while sitting in the back of a police patrol car, her children huddled around her, or from the lobby of the SafePlace Resource Center, located across a parking lot and through multiple security zones, but she must personally reach out and request assistance.

Many women are brought to the shelter by police. Or they are referred by physicians, emergency-room staff, or labor and delivery nurses. Or they may have been told to make the call by child protective workers, or referred by another criminal-justice or social-service agency. Most often, however, the woman herself initiates the call. Like me, she may have carried a "palm card" in her purse for months or years prior to working up the courage or recognizing that she could no longer keep herself or her children safe.

The first question a caller will be asked is, "Are you in a safe place? Is it safe for you to talk?" Contrary to popular belief, women more frequently call during the day when their partner is away than at night or on weekends when they are usually in the most danger but cannot safely make a call without risking further wrath from their abusers. From personal experience I know that it is virtually impossible to make a call for assistance when in the midst of a violent attack. If a caller states that she is *not* in a safe place, she will be asked to quickly hang up the phone and call 911.

Safety Planning First

If the caller is in a safe place and able to talk, the hotline worker will begin by discussing safety planning with her. Together, they will problem solve about all of the ways in which she might be able to keep herself and her children safe.

In preparation for a violent incident she will be told to always know where her purse and keys are located, to tell friends or neighbors about the violence so they can call 911 if they hear suspicious activity coming from the house, to teach the children to call 911 if needed, and to have a safe place she can move to in her home that will present the lowest risk. She will be counseled to avoid areas that are near weapons or without access to an outside door.

Phones and computers should be used with extreme care. I have known several women who have been clandestinely tracked and spied on through hidden tapes and spyware. Several years ago a tape recorder was found in the attic of a woman in my community who was murdered by her husband. The device was connected to her phone, and the brutal homicide was completely captured on tape as she tried to call for help while fighting frantically for her life. Her estranged husband, by fanatically tracking his former wife's activities, had virtually assured his own conviction for murder.

If preparing to leave, the woman will be encouraged to find someone who can keep money, extra clothes, important documents, and an extra set of keys. She will be told to think about opening her own savings account and to think about someone who might be able to lend her money or let her stay with them if necessary. She will be encouraged to rehearse her escape plan. When leaving, she should take the following with her: identification for herself, her and her children's birth certificates, Social Security cards, school and vaccination records, credit cards, keys, driver's license, money, checkbook, ATM card, medication, work permits and green card (if applicable), passport, divorce papers, medical records, lease, house deed, mortgage, insurance papers, address book, pictures, jewelry, children's favorite toys, items of sentiment, and small saleable items.

If they're employed outside the home, most women cannot just quit their jobs, making safety planning at work critical. However, every battered woman must decide on her own if and when she will tell others that her partner has battered her and that she may be at continued risk. She should consider informing supervisors and coworkers of the situation. At times she may decide that reporting the abuse would put her job at risk. If so, she should trust her instincts, but also consider whether there might be a coworker she can confide in and ask for help to screen her calls. Is there someone whom she might ask to provide a safe escort for her while she's going to and from work? She will be encouraged to vary her routes in order to avoid problems from a partner who is familiar with her routine.

If she will be staying in her home, she will be counseled to change her locks, to replace wooden doors with metal doors, and to install a security system, including additional locks, window bars, peepholes, etc. Again, she will be encouraged to teach children how to call 911 and to inform friends and neighbors that her partner no longer lives with her and that the police should be called if he is observed near her home.

A telephone is an essential lifeline. Now many shelters have easy access to donated cell phones, but in the past SafePlace regularly paid to connect phone service for women leaving the shelter. A resident with a donated cell phone programmed to call 911 reinforced the importance of having this lifeline when she went to Houston for a court proceeding. Following the proceeding she stopped at a grocery store, where she realized that her husband was following her. She ran to the back of the store, hid in a walk-in refrigerator, and called 911 to report violation of an existing protective order. Her husband was picked up and jailed.

⌁ Orders of Protection

A final important aspect of safety planning is a protective order. Depending on the state, the document may be called by another name, such as restraining order, but the purpose is always to legally prevent one person from contacting or coming around another. If a woman doesn't already have a protective order, she should be counseled about how to obtain one. If she has one, she should know where the physical document is at all times. Copies of her protective order should be distributed where she lives, works, or visits frequently. Others should know that she has a protective order in effect. If the order is violated, the police and court should be immediately notified, and if the police do not help, she should contact the police department to file a complaint.

It is critical to know that *protective orders are not bulletproof vests, nor do they ensure twenty-four-hour security*. Issuance of a protective order will provide law enforcement and the courts with documentation of abuse and support for the victim when it is violated. However, if an offender is intent on harming his partner, a protective order is not a shield that can ensure her physical safety.

⌁ Safety Planning and Children

When children are involved, as they quite often are, safety issues immediately become immensely more complex. Mothers are encouraged to inform caretakers or teachers about the situation and provide them with copies of protective orders. However, it may be impossible to sufficiently protect a child while he or she is enrolled in a public school or a child-care center.

The inability to protect a child while in school was dramatically underscored several years ago when a mom and her grade-school-age son were admitted to the SafePlace shelter before we had built an on-site school. The son was present when his father had killed another man, his ex-wife's boyfriend, and the son was the one person who could testify to his father's guilt. As the legal father of the boy, the father had rights by law to be notified if his son was enrolled in a local school district. Everyone involved—the mother, the boy, the prosecutors, the shelter staff, and even school representatives—felt the boy's life was at risk if the father found him. Even though the father didn't know to which city his son and ex-wife had fled, we simply could not take the risk of the father tracking his son through his enrollment in a public school, and the family couldn't be relocated far away to another state because they were involved in the ongoing criminal proceedings. So with little other recourse, a private tutor was hired to teach the son within the confines of our facility for months. The father was eventually convicted and sent to prison, freeing the ex-wife and son from the virtual prison they had lived in during the investigation and prosecution of the homicide case.

Even when a school or child-care program has orders in place to prevent release of a child to an abusive parent, it is often difficult or impossible to prevent a determined parent from taking a child. Although this is becoming increasingly less true, in general our schools and child-care programs are not designed as prisons to keep kids in and everyone else out.

While I was working at the Developmental Preschool and Day Care, in Laramie, Wyoming, I had the agonizing responsibility of going to a mother's home to tell her that her estranged husband had just come to the center and taken away their three-year-old twins. Short of lying down behind his pickup truck as he pulled out of the parking lot, there was little I could do to stop his absconding with the children. We called

911 in an attempt to keep him from taking his children, but he literally walked onto the playground and took them. This experience, probably more than any other, convinced me of the need for a school and child-care facility on the secure premises of the shelter. Luckily, in this case the children were returned to their mother within twenty-four hours. Many situations don't have such happy endings.

Once safety planning has been completed, and if the shelter is full, the woman may be assisted by the hotline worker to explore alternatives. Does she have friends or family she can stay with? Is a homeless shelter an alternative? Might she be able to relocate to a battered-women's shelter outside of her community? Is her partner in jail and is she safe until his release? Or can the shelter help her to find financial assistance for a hotel?

Admission to the Shelter

I believe the primary goal of every battered-women's shelter should be how to screen people in, rather than how to screen them out. Our goal should be about how to get to "yes," often a difficult goal given the demand for our services.

At SafePlace we would sometimes assess it to be imperative that a family be admitted to the emergency shelter immediately upon request. Generally, these are families that are brought in by law enforcement. If the shelter is full, space may be made by opening up a meeting room, doubling up families in a room, moving a family into a hotel, or whatever option the shelter staff can conceive. Usually the family is admitted on an emergency basis, giving the woman and the shelter staff time to determine the next steps for trying to ensure the family's safety. This might mean that space will be found in another nearby shelter the next day, the partner may be picked up and taken to jail, or the woman may make arrangements with family and friends who live elsewhere.

However, as I have stated, almost every shelter operates under its own guidelines, policies, and restrictions. What works in one community may be handled differently in another community. And the challenges are usually unique to a specific locale. In Wyoming, geographical barriers are a major consideration — mountain passes close for months in the winter, making towns that are an hour's drive apart in the summer months six or more hours apart during the long winters. The population of Alaska is so sparse that rather than sending cabs for women, shelters there are often forced to transport them by small bush plane from their tiny remote outposts. While waiting, the family may be housed in the local jail.

Unfortunately, there is no guarantee or mandate that says shelter must be available when someone needs it. I know of no program in the United States that is fully funded by public dollars to address community demand; still, despite lack of adequate funding, every shelter works creatively to ensure a family's safety.

Communal Living

Staying in a battered-women's shelter can be comforting, soothing, inspiring, and healing. It may be the first time a mom and her kids have ever felt safe together, the first time they have been able to share the secrets they have lived with. Yet living in a shelter also has its challenges, and some people are simply not a fit. Most programs limit admission to victims of intimate-partner violence, and many are not able to accommodate battered men. In addition, because of the communal nature of many facilities, they may not be able to take mothers with teenage boys. The bathrooms are often set up similar to those in dormitories, with multiple toilets, sinks, and showers in a single room. An individual must be eighteen years old or an emancipated minor to qualify for shelter admission without an accompanying parent or guardian.

In addition, communal living is really difficult for most adults, and some people should not live in shelter because they might pose a potential threat to other residents. If someone is acting out physically, is verbally assaulting others, or is a danger to themselves, there are usually more-appropriate placements. Many people find the loud and often chaotic environment overwhelming.

Most programs will ask residents to help with chores at the shelter in addition to caring for themselves and their children. These are generally typical household chores like cleaning the refrigerator or mopping the floor, and they are assigned or chosen on a rotating basis. It is also a mother's job to care for her children, just as it is when she is in her own home.

Sheltering Women and Children with Multiple Issues

When I began working at what was then the Center for Battered Women, in Austin, the guidelines for admission adhered rigidly to the strict guidelines as set out by the Texas Department of Human Services (TDHS). TDHS, a state grant program, provided approximately 50 percent of the funding to operate the shelter facility and required that we anonymously report in-depth information about the families we served. We had to raise the other 50 percent of our funding, which, I explained to the staff, gave us a great deal of latitude in whom we served, a latitude we needed because abuse isn't limited to mom-and-pop families with 2.5 children.

We have struggled to ensure safety for a transgender woman in the middle of the sex-change process. Her abusive partner had been paying for the surgery and hormone treatments, and if these had been abruptly discontinued, it could have caused serious health issues for the woman. We found a donor willing to help pay for continuing her hormone treatments until she could safely move on.

We have sheltered elderly women who have been terribly abused by their adult children, both male and female. We have sheltered a homeless woman who was brutally gang-raped by a group of men in her encampment. We have sheltered a young woman who witnessed a gang murder and was in need of sanctuary. We regularly provide shelter for gay men abused by their male partners as well as heterosexual men abused by their wives. And, of course, SafePlace shelters recent rape survivors who don't feel safe to return to their homes.

Battered women are people first, and they can display all the faults and foibles of the human species. We deal with women who are enormously caring and generous, and we deal with those who have tempers, who lie, and who may cheat and hurt others. Women come into a shelter with all of the baggage and messes we all carry around.

Shelter personnel will always consider the safety and needs of the shelter community, as well as that of an individual. It was heartbreaking to realize we couldn't safely shelter a woman who had a teenage son with a developmental disability because he acted out sexually with younger children, mirroring the sexual abuse perpetrated against him by his father. Our first responsibility had to be to the safety of the full community.

Given the high incidence of mental illness and substance abuse co-occurring with domestic violence, SafePlace, like every shelter, is often faced with dealing with a client who has multiple and disruptive issues. Like most battered-women's shelters, SafePlace has struggled mightily to figure out how to serve women who abuse drugs, sell their bodies, or are at times harmful to their own children. If we have witnessed or been told of abuse against a child, then we must, by law, report the abuse to Child Protective Services. If a woman is actively abusing drugs or alcohol, she will not be allowed to use substances while at the shelter and will be encouraged and assisted to engage in a treatment program. Shelter staff also work closely with local mental-health programs in order to attempt to address psychological needs. Affordable psychiatric services are often particularly difficult to access, necessitating creative advocacy on the part of shelter staff and volunteers.

Clearly, forced participation in the sex trade is often an extension of domestic violence and must be acknowledged and treated as such by battered-women's advocates. However, it can be difficult to provide emergency shelter for women engaged in the sex trade, even while acknowledging that they are indeed victims of domestic abuse. Many shelters exclude sex workers altogether, judging them as prostitutes rather than battered women. However, I believe they should be treated like any other victim of abuse. Continued participation in the sex trade, an illegal activity, may preclude their continued stay in an emergency battered-women's shelter, but a woman should not be judged guilty before the fact because of prior coerced behavior.

Shelter for People with Specific Ethnicities, Religions, or Disabilities

Many large communities have created special shelter programs that directly target specific populations. Shelter programs operate in various cities for Asian, South Asian, and Pacific Islander populations, as well as for people who are deaf or hearing impaired, or are members of certain religious faiths, particularly Islam. At SafePlace we took the somewhat unorthodox approach of helping to mentor and grow these programs as a part of our services. If by helping to develop these programs we are able to more effectively serve a broader cross-section of our community, the better we will have met our mission of ending rape, sexual abuse, and domestic violence.

Often, these programs have operated as separate nonprofit organizations with the support and assistance of SafePlace. Rather than creating their own emergency shelter programs, these partner agencies send their clients to the SafePlace shelter when necessary, while providing their own supportive services. Saheli, an Austin agency designed to help and empower Asian victims and survivors of domestic abuse by providing them access to services and by increasing community awareness, has worked hand in hand with SafePlace since its inception. Rather than creating a separate emergency shelter, Saheli provides services in cooperation with SafePlace.

Services for the deaf and hard of hearing were originally provided through a partnership with DAWCAS, the Deaf and Abused Women's and Children's Advocacy Services, until the agency was dissolved and SafePlace stepped in to fill the void.

Building a Shelter from the Ground Up

When, in 2000, Austin's SafePlace had the opportunity to design and build a new shelter from the ground up, we created a facility that tried to be welcoming and accessible to people with all types of disabilities, as well as to men, rape survivors, and others with special needs. Prior to building, we spent months touring other facilities, talking with people from across the nation about what worked and what didn't, and conducting focus groups with former clients, staff, children, and volunteers.

Not surprisingly, former residents of shelter recommended that safety be the highest priority. Former residents told us, "We want it to look forbidding from the outside, to give a 'don't come in here' message to batterers. Then as soon as we drive in, it should be welcoming."

Shelter clients wanted control — they wanted their power back — and they wanted to prove to themselves and their kids that they were competent, even about the most basic things like preparing their own meals. Moms wanted to be able to cook for themselves and their children when, how, and what they wanted. They told us to put the laundry room in the most accessible site in the building and to make it a location where they could do their wash while also watching their children play. Having some control over the temperature in their own space was essential. Women also wanted to have easy access to the outside from their living quarters. By giving women added control over their environment, cultural preferences could be observed, thereby making the shelter a more comfortable place for everyone.

During the designing and building of the new shelter, our team included Gil Crane, long-time facilities manager for SafePlace, who consistently advocated for low maintenance and durability. Diane McDaniel Rhodes, shelter director at the time, took into account every possible safety and security consideration, as well as programming components and space utilization. Julia Spann, then deputy director of programs, conducted the initial client focus groups and managed the finances, and Wendie Abramson, director of disabilities services, ensured that we built a facility accessible to all.

I was the relentless voice of frugality. My constant refrain was, "I'm not going to pay for that." At one point the architect became so frustrated with me that he said he would personally pick up the extra expense for something he considered to be critically important to the esthetics of the building. I let him. I was also working to raise the millions of dollars needed to build the facility and then sustain its operation.

Each of these issues was critical to designing and building a model shelter program for battered women and their children that would sustain SafePlace families well into the twenty-first century.

I cannot overstate the importance of safety. Everything must be considered — from how to design playgrounds to how to keep unwanted people out without any unsupervised spaces. The children who come into a shelter have seen or experienced violence in their homes, and many have been sexually molested. They may try to act out their own experiences with other children, and it is our responsibility to guard against any situations that might allow children to be violated by their friends and classmates.

Diane attended to many details, such as making sure there were no drop-down ceilings in private areas because they would allow an easy hiding place for contraband like drugs or weapons. She helped to figure out how to build multiple kitchens for use by the clients that would also be approved by the fire marshal. She saw to it that each bedroom door had a combination key lock that could be reprogrammed as old clients moved out and new ones moved in, ensuring each family a private and secure space of its own.

Each family's private space usually consisted of one private bedroom with a Hollywood-style bath. Each bedroom included a sink, and there was a lockable door to a shared toilet and bath/shower situated between two bedrooms. If a family were particularly large, they might be assigned two bedrooms. Each family was also assigned a locked drawer or shelf in the kitchen, made from heavy-gauge, steel-wire mesh. This allowed contents to be visible, the shelf to be easily cleaned, and each family to address its own special dietary needs and wants.

One of our many challenges was to build a facility that could house more than a hundred people, but to do so in a way that created a sense of community for the families living there. We heard over and over that having the chance to connect with other women in an informal and unsupervised atmosphere — like the kitchen table at the SAFE Project shelter in Laramie, Wyoming, was for me — could often be the lifeline that helps a woman understand she is not alone and that she can create a different and better life. We ultimately decided to build six smaller shelters — what we referred to as "clusters" — within one big facility. Each cluster consists of a family/living area with an attached kitchen, a screened outdoor porch, and five bedrooms, one of which has a private bathroom that is fully wheelchair accessible. The building is two stories, with three clusters on each floor.

An additional guest suite was built to accommodate an individual or family with special needs, such as a recent rape survivor, a man, or someone with special health needs. The guest suite is similar to a studio apartment, with a small kitchen, bath, and bedroom area. The need for such a space had been underscored many times over the years.

⌁ Shelter Space for Children

A critically important part of any battered-women's shelter is the space created for children, both indoors and out. Since we were designing and building a new facility, we had the luxury of creating specific spaces for teens and young children, as well as a computer lab where volunteers could help children and moms learn computer skills and the children could utilize the computers for homework. As described earlier, thanks to generous donors we were also able to build a separate school and child-care center on the premises. This facility was built across the parking lot but totally within the confines of the shelter's security, allowing for the emotional and physical separation associated with going to school but still ensuring safety for the attendees. Three different playgrounds and a basketball/play court are incorporated within the boundaries of the shelter premises.

⌁ Food, Clothing, and Other Necessities

We were able to create a commissary that operates much like a convenience store. It is stocked with staples such as milk, eggs, flour, cheese, and canned goods, all provided to the residents free of charge. The commissary goes through an astonishing amount of food for the twenty-five to thirty-plus families that are in residence on any given day.

Most women come into shelter with several very young children, even babies, and all of the associated accoutrement. We had to build one entire room just to store car seats. There is little that brings home the reality of the numbers of children living in a battered-women's shelter more than looking at stacked rows of dozens of well-worn infant and toddler car seats.

Most families arrive at the shelter with little except the clothes they are wearing. Staff and volunteers, with the assistance of the community, set about trying to provide all of the many necessities of life, the numbers of which are often staggering. At SafePlace, we regularly asked generous donors to help replenish these consumables on a regular basis: items like 200 to 400 diapers a day, 1,825 boxes of baby wipes each year, 45 gallons of milk and 35 loaves of bread each week, 10 rolls of paper towels and 4 to 5 dozen eggs each day, and almost 3,000 toothbrushes each year. Women are also given items like blankets and pillows to take with them when they leave the shelter. At SafePlace, we planned to go through 49 sets of sheets and 91 sets of towels each week, over 2,000 pillows a year, and 5 blankets each day. When people from the community would say to me, "If there's anything I can do to help, please don't hesitate to ask," I always took them at their word. We developed relationships with egg farmers who weekly delivered 30 dozen fresh eggs to our door at no charge, small businesses that donated a palette of diapers every month, and bakeries that provided fresh bread each day.

Shelter and Pets

Pets are yet another thing that battered women are often forced to leave at home when fleeing an abusive partner. Prior to our having children, Jay knew he could keep me in check and in his control by holding my dog, Billy, hostage. I remember standing in the street outside my house, afraid to go back in, but also unwilling to leave because Jay was standing at the door holding my shaking, frightened dog, telling me I would never see Billy alive again if I left.

Those of us with pets can no more imagine leaving our innocent, vulnerable dog or cat behind to be brutalized than we can imagine leaving our children behind. Rarely do battered-women's shelters allow pets in the facility. However, many, like SafePlace, work with volunteers and community organizations to provide foster care for the animal while the family is in the shelter.

Maintaining a Safe and Secure Shelter Facility

As you can see, creating and running shelter facilities for battered women and their children involves numerous complex problems, one of the most important of which is security. Figuring out the security for the SafePlace campus was a true puzzler given the number of facilities that would be included. Besides the shelter, school, and child-care buildings, all of which require extensive security in order to keep batterers from getting in, we also had a transitional-housing apartment complex where families lived and worked for up to eighteen months, and a resource center that housed the organization's administrative offices as well as most of the nonresident services like individual and group counseling. All of this involved hundreds of people coming and going each month.

Contrary to what some people may believe, battered-women's shelters are not prisons — they are not built or designed to keep anyone in the facility who doesn't want to stay there. Rather, they are designed and built to keep people on the outside from getting in unless they have been specifically invited. Many times over the years I have fielded requests from different entities about taking in a woman and keeping her from getting out: "She will try to return to her husband, but you can't let her." The concern is almost always valid and caring, but *battered-women's shelters are not designed or prepared to protect people who don't want protecting.*

While trying to figure out the dilemma of security, I landed on the idea of asking retired Secret Service personnel if they would consider consulting with us. After all, who would be more knowledgeable about solving complex security issues than the people charged with protecting the president of the United States? And I had just the person to ask for help. Luci Baines Johnson, daughter of the thirty-sixth president, Lyndon Baines Johnson, has served on the SafePlace Foundation Board of Trustees for many years. Her mother and father had retired to Austin, bringing a cadre of Secret Service personnel with them, most of whom also retired in the area.

When Luci put out the word asking for their help, several stepped forward, giving assistance and advice on how to make security an integral part of the design of the entire campus while creating a unified system operating at many different levels. Even with the pro-bono assistance of the retired Secret Service agents, the cost of the extensive security systems was great. However, the Meadows Foundation, located in Dallas, understood the need and awarded a grant that substantially paid for the work.

Traditionally, battered-women's shelters have relied on the secrecy of their locations as their first line of safety; if a batterer doesn't know where the shelter is located, then he won't be able to find his wife. Even residents were held to an incredibly high standard of secrecy, jeopardizing their continued stay at the shelter if they told anyone of its location without prior permission. This policy existed despite the fact that many people in the community already knew exactly where SafePlace was.

However, as the new SafePlace campus grew in size, it became apparent that we were fooling ourselves if we believed we were maintaining a confidential location. The site is situated across the street from a city golf course, and players regularly asked about the large, fenced compound. And most cab drivers and law enforcement officers knew the purpose of the building at which they dropped off women and children carrying their belongings in paper bags.

We finally recognized that it was time to question our deeply held conviction that the location of a battered-women's shelter should always be kept confidential. Might we actually enhance security by letting go of the illusion that no one knew where the facility was located? Working with a group of staff, volunteers, former clients, board members, and advisors from the community, including the sheriff and other law enforcement officers, we carefully examined the idea of lifting the veil of confidentiality of the location. How might we be able to maintain and possibly even enhance the safety of our residents by doing so?

We eventually decided that we could, in fact, improve safety by acknowledging the reality that we no longer operated a confidential location. It was time for us to create procedures and systems that supported this fact rather than trying to pretend otherwise. All SafePlace employees are now trained in extensive security procedures to which everyone strictly adheres, and the shelter continues to be one of the most secure anywhere in the nation.

Dropping the illusion of secrecy had another important impact: It reduced the shame and stigma that some women feel when they go to shelter. Secrecy is a tactic used by batterers to maintain control, and battered women and their children are forced to carry the family secrets. Coming to a confidential shelter reinforces the concept that domestic violence is a secret family problem when, in fact, it is a community problem and all of us can play a part in keeping a family safe. Secrets often equal shame in people's opinions. We try to instill in a battered victim the idea that she doesn't need to keep yet another secret or to be ashamed of coming to shelter. The person who hurt her is the one operating under the cloak of secrets and shame; she doesn't have to.

We wouldn't recommend this approach for all shelters. If a program doesn't have strong support from local law enforcement, the ability to invest in security technology, and the time and resources to develop and provide security training for staff, then ensuring a secret location is important. SafePlace was fortunate enough to be able to build a shelter that corresponded to the values and philosophies we held dear: domestic violence shouldn't be a secret family matter.

Empowering Women to Help Themselves

Most domestic-violence programs operate from an empowerment model: helping to provide women with the education and resources to help themselves. Being battered or assaulted is an event or life circumstance; it is not what defines a woman. What anyone needs to cope with violence in an intimate relationship is unique to that person. Those of us who have done this work have been privileged to meet and live with the individuals who seek and obtain shelter; we learn as much from them as they learn from us.

Again, programs operate differently all across the nation. Some agencies are 100 percent operated and staffed by volunteers, while others may function as a small program within a larger, more diverse agency. But in some form or fashion most women entering a shelter are assigned an advocate or case manager (terminology varies from shelter to shelter), whether it's a volunteer or paid staff member. The advocate is charged with helping the resident to develop goals and action steps for being able to move safely from the shelter.

Yes, the number-one goal for every family entering a battered-women's shelter is how to move safely out of the shelter—a goal that is often much easier said than done.

One of the first questions people ask about a shelter is, "How long do you allow women to stay?" Permissible length of stay is specific to each shelter program. At SafePlace, women are given a few days of "respite," time to begin to heal and refocus their energy, prior to beginning to work toward leaving. As long as a woman is doing what she needs to do to try to proactively build toward a safer life, she will not be forced to leave. However, everyone is acutely aware that the longer a woman and her children stay at the shelter, the fewer people we are able to let in on the front end—which may translate into fewer lives saved.

The advocate will work with the woman to address both criminal and civil legal needs; this may involve everything from attaining a divorce, to obtaining a protective order, to testifying in criminal proceedings against a former partner. She will help with ensuring that the family's health-care needs are met and the children's immunizations are current, and that the family is enrolled in any health-insurance programs for which they are eligible. Safe and affordable housing is one of the biggest obstacles families usually face: Housing that is affordable is often not safe. I cannot tell you how many women I have talked to over the years who have told me they are returning to their batterer because "he doesn't hit the children, and at least they are able to live in a safe neighborhood where they aren't afraid to go outside." Transitional-housing programs, like that built and operated by SafePlace, while enormously successful in meeting the stated goal of achieving economic and emotional independence for residents, are expensive to operate. Many cities don't even have such programs available. Those that do exist can usually accept only a minimal percentage of the families trying to get in—almost always, "the inn is full."

The advocate will also help the woman and her children understand what it means to live in a cooperative residential environment. Prejudices must be left on the other side of the gate—black, brown, white, young, old, gay, straight, Jewish, Muslim, Christian, and everyone in between must live together and respect one another.

When I first took the helm at what was then the Center for Battered Women, all shelter residents took part in mandatory counseling as a condition of their continued stay. I strongly felt this mandate was in opposition to a model of empowerment and self-determination, and I worked to change the policy. At SafePlace, all shelter residents can now participate in therapeutic counseling if they want, but it is never a mandate for continued services. When counseling was a requirement for staying at the shelter, clients complained bitterly about being forced into it, but once the requirement was lifted and counseling became voluntary, many women chose to participate. Most often, a client's primary need is for advocacy to address basic needs, safety planning, and education about the cycle of violence. Therapy may come later—after they have stabilized and left shelter.

Defining Success

How does one define the success of a shelter program? I am repeatedly asked how we "make sure the women don't return to their batterers." But should success only be defined by ensuring that a woman never returns to her batterer? Or can success be defined by a woman learning how to keep herself and her children safe, even though she may choose to return to her abusive partner? Yes, many women return to a shelter time and time again—should we judge them as "failures"? I think not.

Susan and her son returned to the SafePlace shelter eleven times in nine years. Her son was twelve years old the last time they came. Had she not had the shelter to go to, might she have died during one of her husband's attacks? And what of her son, the little boy who because of his frequents stays at a battered-women's shelter began to learn about a new kind of relationship and a different way of interacting? Many who evaluate domestic-violence programs only on the basis of leaving and staying away from an abusive marriage might have judged this small family a "failure." I would disagree; rather, Susan learned ways to keep herself and her son alive.

10

beyond shelter

You have facilitated our gaining skills that have empowered us to take charge of our own lives, to be in control of our own destinies, and to evolve into the people we want to be. You have provided us with a forum to air our beliefs, thoughts, and feelings without having to worry about being judged, abused, or argued with. You have helped us to learn new ways to view ourselves, the people we love, and the world around us. These points of view may not always have been the most pleasant, or what we wanted to see, but they have always brought us back to the same basic premise: we are phenomenal women! You have helped us learn to love each other and to love ourselves.

You have done all of these things not only for us, but with us, and with great humor, empathy, kindness, and love.

— A supportive-housing and life-skills graduate

S USAN, FIRST MENTIONED IN CHAPTER 9, HAD BEEN IN OUR shelter eleven times in nine years. The last time she was admitted her husband had been beating her with a baseball bat until her twelve-year-old son intervened, stepping in front of his father and begging him to stop.

Susan was similar to so many battered women. She was in her mid-thirties and had been with her husband since she was young. Short and a little pudgy, she bought most of her clothes from Goodwill or the local discount store and cut her hair herself. She had no high-school diploma and no viable job skills other than working at less than minimum wage as a waitress at lunch counters or as a motel maid. After one violent incident her manager at a restaurant told her not to return to work because her black eyes and bruises were off-putting to the customers — "not very appetizing," her boss said. Another time, she tried to continue working as a maid at a motel while staying at the shelter, only to learn that her husband had convinced another worker to let him into a room she was scheduled to clean. He surprised her when she entered the room, beat her, and made her quit her job and return home with him.

Following one of her earlier shelter stays, she had moved with her son into an apartment completely outfitted with donated furniture. However, she was unable to keep up the rent and utility payments, and her electricity was soon shut off. Facing eviction, she called her husband and asked him to take her back. Prior to allowing her to return to their home he broke all of her new furniture into splintered bits.

Despite repeated efforts to get away from her abusive husband, Susan always ended up returning to him because she simply could not support herself and her son on her own. However, during her eleventh stay at the shelter, SafePlace was preparing to open its new supportive-housing apartment community. Susan and her son were the first clients admitted to the program, and to this day I know of no better example of the importance of comprehensive services beyond shelter.

Susan and her son moved out of the emergency shelter and into a two-bedroom apartment within hours of our receiving a certificate of occupancy. Each building was filled with families within days. Local churches and other organizations adopted families and helped to provide them with furniture, linens, and housewares. We abandoned our initial idea of asking different interior designers and furniture stores to decorate apartments when we realized that each family would likely be starting their new home from scratch and would need to take all their belongings with them when they moved on, putting us in the difficult position of constantly recruiting designers and stores to decorate the apartments as new families moved in. We also realized that women would want to choose their own décor in what was, for many, their first real home.

Susan was delighted with her new home, and her joy was infectious and apparent to everyone. She regularly allowed interested donors and groups to tour what she considered her palace. I particularly remember a Saturday when Susan helped me to conduct a tour for a small group. That morning I had stopped at an ATM with my daughter Megan in tow to withdraw $100. Megan had stared wide-eyed at the crisp $20 bills and said, "Mom, we're rich."

"No," I responded, "this is just to get us through the weekend. We are certainly not rich."

Later that afternoon, as I stood with Susan in the small courtyard outside the front door of the first safe place she had called home in decades, a woman touring the facility asked Susan how she supported herself financially. Susan, always open and honest, responded cheerily, "I get $170 a month in public assistance for myself and my son."

I went home to my daughter that afternoon and said, "Megan, you're right — we are rich."

Susan was luckier than most families living on the same amount of assistance because her rent was based on a sliding scale, allowing her to pay a minimal amount for housing. But from that $170 she still had to pay for utilities, phone, food, and clothing. She and her son tended to eat whatever special donations the local food bank had received that month.

Despite these hardships Susan was extraordinarily rich in spirit and will. Within weeks she had successfully completed a course for her high-school general equivalency diploma (GED) and passed the test. She then enrolled in classes at the community college located across the street from her apartment. She also advocated with the school district to successfully get the bus stop for her son moved closer to their home, explaining that she continued to have concerns about their safety. She energetically participated in life skills training and counseling, as did her son. When her son made the honor roll at his new school, for the first time ever in his life, he proudly presented the certificate to his SafePlace counselor, and said, "We did this together."

Susan and her son stayed in supportive housing for eighteen months. When they moved, it was into another apartment where Susan was hired as the manager. She continued her studies at the community college. Not only was she able to live free from the beatings she had endured so regularly in her marriage, her son was also able to break the cycle of abuse for future generations.

As Susan's story so perfectly demonstrates, for many women and children emergency shelter is simply not enough. In order to become truly independent economically and emotionally, women need legal services, transitional and permanent housing, child care, education, job training, life skills training, and therapeutic counseling. Particularly for women living in poverty, stopping physical violence is not always their number-one priority. They say, "I can deal with the violence, but I'm not going to put my kids on the street." Rather than just offering a formula for leaving an abusive relationship, we should be asking what services women need in order to become economically secure. Many of these services are available to some limited degree in most communities, but seldom can a person fully access all of them. The systems are simply underfunded and overloaded, and they vary widely from city to city and state to state. There is no one call to make, or place to go, for a woman to get help in dealing with these concerns. My best advice is to call the National Domestic Violence Hotline at (800) 799-7233 (799-SAFE; website www.ndvh.org) and ask about resources available in your community.

Supportive-Housing Programs

As demonstrated again and again, it is impossible to overstate the importance of safe, affordable housing for battered women and their children.

In a twenty-five-city survey conducted in 2003 by the US Conference of Mayors, domestic violence was ranked as the number-one cause of homelessness in 44 percent of the cities surveyed. National research and our own experience demonstrate that domestic violence, homelessness, and poverty go hand in hand. If our goal as individuals and a society is to end domestic violence, it is imperative that we end the dangerous cycle of abuse, shelter, poverty, homelessness, and ultimately hopelessness.

Many battered-women's programs now operate or work cooperatively with supportive-housing programs, which provide an interim place for women and their children to live while they work toward making the transition from emergency shelter to a positive, permanent living environment and a life of self-sufficiency. But make no mistake, these programs are expensive to develop and operate, and in recent years essential governmental support and funding have decreased.

The three core elements of supportive housing are an affordable place to live, support service programs, and the creation of community for families previously isolated by homelessness and domestic violence. In the SafePlace program, every resident is carefully screened and signs a lease that includes working with a case manager toward achieving goals for independence.

At SafePlace we decided to take a whole-family approach to the design and implementation of the services associated with supportive housing. The entire intact family, both adults and children, are engaged in the program. Additionally, each individual in the family is considered from a "whole person" perspective by looking at their entire history, not just an isolated incident of violence or a single environmental element. Intensive attention is given to the multiple issues or problems in the residents' current life and past history, and to how these issues impact their lives and their relationships to their family.

As SafePlace's supportive-housing program has evolved, it has ended up serving women who have very few options and who encounter multiple barriers to violence-free lives. This makes the whole-person philosophy critically important when considered in the context of the average resident. She is a woman who is estranged from her family of origin, often a graduate of the foster-care system, a survivor of childhood sexual or physical abuse, and a victim of long-term battering or multiple battering relationships. Almost always, the children in the family have been victims of physical, and quite often sexual, abuse, in addition to having witnessed violence in their homes. These families are almost always desperately poor. Many also have immigration issues, little education, and mental-health or substance-abuse problems.

Notably, supportive housing is not a shelter; nor is it a permanent living arrangement or an institutionalized facility. Many supportive-housing programs are dispersed throughout a broad area and incorporate a variety of housing types. SafePlace built a single apartment complex on its thirteen-acre campus. The entire supportive-housing complex has its own security system, in addition to being incorporated into the overall SafePlace security structure.

In our initial plans for the supportive-housing community we had decided against including security measures beyond what would be found in an average apartment complex. Our rationale was that if more intensive security were required, the families should be in the shelter. However, as women applied for admission to supportive housing, we fairly quickly began to recognize the problem with our plan. Many of the families seeking admission continued to be in extremely dangerous situations. One woman's husband had driven her across the border into Mexico, slit her throat, and thrown her out of the car to die on the side of the road. She lived and was eventually transferred to the SafePlace shelter because he had not been apprehended. Another woman's husband had repeatedly attempted to kidnap their baby. He, too, had never been apprehended. Admission to supportive housing would allow these women to pay for rent and child care on a sliding scale, and to obtain financial assistance to help pay for educational and job-training programs.

As I listened to their stories I realized how unfair it would be if these women were yet again denied what was best for them because their lives continued to be controlled, even if indirectly, by their abusive husbands. I decided that we simply could not let the batterer win once again, so intensive security plans, procedures, and structures were quickly initiated and installed.

Many transitional-housing programs operated by domestic-violence agencies have opted not to provide the kind of intensive security Safe-Place has chosen to incorporate into its facilities. However, it was the right decision for SafePlace, and the wisdom of our decision, given that the housing is located on the SafePlace campus, has been reinforced repeatedly over the years.

Beyond a place to live, the second core element of supportive housing is social services that offer the types of programs residents need to create stable, safe, self-sufficient lives. Social services may be provided through partnerships, collaborations, and the sponsoring agency. They generally include case management, counseling, life-skills training, children's therapeutic and recreational services, legal representation, health services, substance-abuse treatment, child-support services, job training, immigration assistance, child care, and some kind of follow-up support once the client has moved from the transitional-housing apartment. Through a combination of both internal services and external partnerships, clients are able to successfully transition from emergency shelter to permanent housing.

An important but little-understood aspect of supportive housing is life-skills training. Many residents have never had a bank account in their own name, balanced a checkbook, put together a household budget, utilized public transportation, or mastered many other basic skills of everyday life. Classes in résumé writing, interviewing for a job, how to dress for work, employee rights and responsibilities, and tenant rights are offered, often in multiple languages. The range of "life skills" needed to live an independent life is endless, and volunteers from the community can help provide the various types of training. Women benefit from basic auto repair taught by master mechanics, parenting taught by accomplished moms, and nutrition taught by licensed dietitians.

Life-skills training also focuses on building self-esteem and a sense of focus and purpose. Most women in supportive housing have never learned to dream — to expect a better life or to know that they are smart enough and good enough to deserve the best.

The creation of a community is the third and final component of supportive housing. This is where the real and lasting impact of a supportive-housing program lies, because being part of a community provides the opportunity for each resident to benefit from the insights and camaraderie of her peers as she begins to break down the intense isolation perpetuated by domestic violence. It is in the creation of a sense of belonging that each individual has the greatest chance of building life-long friendships and achieving more security and stability.

Supportive-housing programs have only become popular in the last ten to fifteen years. Prior to that, women often had few choices. I am reminded of Rosa, a woman I met who told me of having sought counseling from SafePlace as an adult in order to help her deal with sexual molestation as a child by her stepfather. The story of Rosa's childhood and her mother's lack of choices dramatically demonstrates how families can become trapped in a cycle of abuse because of the nature of poverty and the lack of alternatives for a better life.

Rosa blamed her mother for the abuse perpetrated by her stepfather. In her words, "I felt like my mother sacrificed me for the sake of my brothers." As I talked with her I found I agreed. It did sound as though her mother had sacrificed her for the sake of the rest of the family. But given similar circumstances, what would any of us have done? Rosa's father had deserted the family, including his four sons and one daughter, when the children were quite small. Rosa's mother spoke no English, had no education, and had never held a job outside of the home. As a poor woman with five young children, uneducated and unskilled, Rosa's mother felt lucky to find a man who would even look at her, let alone marry her and take on the care and support of her children. Unfortunately, part of that "care and support" included regular sexual molestation — rape — of her daughter, Rosa, beginning when Rosa was eleven years old and ending only when she moved away from home.

Rosa said she never told anyone what was happening at the time, because she knew that if she did it would tear her family apart. The stepfather was their only means of support. But she also believes that her mother, in some part of herself, knew what was going on and chose not to see it because the resulting consequences would be too devastating for the rest of the family.

This happened over thirty years ago, at a time when society recognized incest even less than now, and there was no such thing as a battered-women's shelter, rape crisis center, or supportive housing. I found myself wondering what else Rosa's mother could have done. Her choices were truly pretty grim.

Rosa confronted her family when her own daughter turned eleven years old and she realized that, in order to protect her daughter as well as her many nieces, she needed to tell what had happened to her. Her step-father denied the abuse, and her mother left him for a short while but has since returned. Two of her four brothers have stood solidly in her support; the other two have been lost to her. In effect, her fears were realized: Her acknowledgment of what happened to her has torn her family apart.

Rosa is doing well. She has never married; nor, according to her, has she maintained any long-term relationships with a man. Instead, she has been fiercely independent. In telling Rosa's story I think it is important to acknowledge her mother's story as well—that of a woman with five young children, deserted by her husband, with no education or job skills, desperate to put a roof over her children's heads. What if Rosa's mother had had a safe place to take her children when her husband abandoned them? What if she'd had the hope of building a new life instead of relying upon the good will and decency of whatever man would take her and her children into his home? What if she'd had a supportive-housing program, like the one available to Susan, and with it the hope of a better life for all of them?

Counseling Programs

Rosa's daughter was spared the damage of childhood sexual abuse because of Rosa's vigilance and her determination that her daughter would have a childhood different from and better than her own. Rosa acknowledges that she found the insight and the courage to confront her family because of counseling she received as an adult. Through counseling, Rosa understood that she was in no way to blame for the sexual assaults, and that she must protect her own daughter.

Therapeutic counseling, an important service associated with supportive housing and emergency shelter, is also valuable for all people dealing with issues of rape, sexual abuse, and domestic violence — even those who may not need housing. Many people, like Rosa, seek counseling years after their experience with sexual or domestic violence. Others seek counseling while staying in the abusive relationship. Many children are referred for counseling because of trauma related to recent abuse.

Unfortunately, like every type of service associated with domestic violence, there are never enough therapists to meet the demand. At SafePlace, as in every other domestic-violence program in the country, nonresident counseling programs always operate with lengthy waiting lists. And although an individual may not be in immediate crisis at the point when they seek counseling, if put on a waiting list, they may not reach out again. Many people can be referred to therapists in the community, but many others cannot afford to pay the market rate for therapy, have no third-party benefits to help pay (such as health insurance or Crime Victims Assistance), or simply would prefer to utilize the counseling service provided through the domestic-violence program.

Several years ago I decided I wanted to better understand who the people on the waiting list were, so I read their intake information. We had a mom with two kids, a six-year-old girl and a four-year-old boy, both of whom had been sexually abused by their father, who also physically abused their mom. Another woman, a mother of three who'd been physically abused by her husband for the previous fourteen years, was referred to SafePlace by the hospital after her husband brought her into the emergency room following a beating. A six-year-old girl also waited to see a counselor. A stranger had tried to force her to perform oral sex. And a young woman self-referred, reporting attacks by her husband that included choking, black eyes, bites, and broken bones.

On that day, in 2002, SafePlace had thirty-two women and one man on the waiting list for nonresident counseling services. An additional ninety-nine children from sixty-one families were on a separate waiting list for children's counseling. It would be nice to think the situation has improved over the last few years, but, in fact, the opposite is true because both state and federal governments have dramatically reduced funding for almost all direct human-service programming.

Although counseling is often considered a "mushy" or "feel-good" service by those who fund battered-women's programs, it is usually essential to the healing process. Women must begin to understand the patterns and behaviors associated with having been a victim. They must learn to quit blaming themselves and how to create empowered lives. It was only after seeking therapy that I began to fully understand and accept some of the patterns of abuse in my own life.

The general community recognizes and knows most domestic-violence agencies for their shelter programs, but in actuality far more women and children are typically seen through nonresident counseling programs. And these programs are much more cost-effective than the relatively expensive shelter or supportive-housing services. If someone can stay safely in their home while dealing through counseling with the issues associated with victimization, it is always considered the first option for service. In addition, a broad cross-section of the community seeks services through nonresident counseling. At SafePlace, agency therapists have counseled executives, physicians, and university professors, as well as young children, adolescents, men, people with disabilities, the transgendered, and people of every nationality, religion, and ethnicity. Counseling is also provided at middle- and high-school campuses for adolescents who have experienced rape, sexual abuse, or domestic violence.

Even though individual and family counseling are available, generally the primary goal is to move clients into a group setting. A person may participate in a group formed specifically for recent rape survivors, say, or adults molested as children, or battered women, but in reality rarely can someone be so neatly categorized; usually she or he has been victimized in multiple ways. So most people self-select the group they feel best meets their needs. A group can help to create an all-important sense of community and to demonstrate to participants that they are not alone and they are not to blame.

Not all domestic-violence programs offer therapeutic counseling with credentialed counseling staff. In addition to the expense of hiring and retaining appropriate staff, some programs espouse the idea that therapeutic counseling runs counter to the belief that battering is not the fault of the victim. However, as I've said, I believe it is imperative to meet a woman where she is, to listen to her, and to try to provide her with the services she feels she needs. And again, drawing on my personal experience and that of the thousands of women I have known and worked with, many battered women request counseling services and need therapeutic intervention in order to recognize the patterns that have kept them enmeshed in abusive relationships and to truly heal.

Additional Services

Most domestic-violence programs also provide assistance and support in addressing the myriad other needs that must be met in order for clients to build safe and secure lives. SafePlace's on-site child-care center is primarily utilized by shelter clients but is also available to supportive-housing residents until they can find safe, affordable child care in the community. Because of the importance of child care and early childhood intervention in the ongoing safety and economic security of moms and children, SafePlace works extensively with multiple community partners to try to ensure that these services are available for all of the women needing them.

Quite often the additional services are provided through collaborative partnerships with other service providers. One of the most important — and most difficult — services to access is civil legal assistance. Getting out of an abusive marriage requires legal assistance, and even if the family has assets, they are often not available to the woman for legal costs or other expenses. District and county attorneys will represent a woman in issues related to an assault or other criminal proceedings, but there is a woeful lack of legal assistance to help with family law, including divorce, child custody, immigration, housing, and other civil issues.

Most battered-women's programs work hand in hand with a local legal-aid program, and thankfully, legal aid usually prioritizes cases involving family violence. Even so, every legal-aid program across the country is understaffed, underfunded, and therefore grievously unable to cope with the volume of cases that come its way.

In addition, most domestic-violence programs work with a cadre of pro-bono attorneys who otherwise specialize in real estate, corporate law, or other areas. These attorneys agree to represent a battered woman at no charge because they know it is a way to give back and to fulfill a part of the altruistic belief in justice and truth that brought them to the practice of law in the beginning. I have repeatedly heard pro-bono lawyers say that these are the most difficult, complex, and time-consuming cases they have ever worked on — as well as the most gratifying and fulfilling.

Advocacy and assistance in navigating the legal system is an essential component of many battered-women's programs. SafePlace placed an advocate at the office of the Travis County attorney almost twenty years ago, thinking the advocate would be able to assist existing clients to obtain protective orders and deal with other legal issues women must address through the criminal-justice system. Much to our surprise and chagrin, we began to see an entirely new population of women — women who had never called the shelter for assistance but had instead sought direct assistance from the legal system. They came in droves every day, asking for help in staying safe. We eventually also placed staff within the district attorney's office and the Austin Police Department. All were overwhelmed by the numbers of families seeking assistance and safety, and astonished at the fact that they were each dealing with completely different populations.

Although most criminal-justice agencies have victim assistance programs in place, the role of the domestic-violence agency staff within these systems is different. The advocate employed by the criminal-justice agency is primarily responsible for assisting the victim as the case is prosecuted. She will have a dual allegiance to helping the victim and the successful outcome of the case. By contrast, the advocate from the battered-women's program should always hold the safety and support of the victim as her primary objective, and sometimes that may mean not going forward with prosecution or being at odds with a determination by the criminal-justice agency.

Battered-women's programs necessarily try to work in partnership with local criminal-justice agencies. We rely on these agencies for protection and assistance, and almost always prefer to embrace common goals rather than taking antagonistic positions. However, that isn't always possible. When the coroner, an arm of the criminal-justice system, declared the death of a young Austin woman named Amanda Smith to be "assisted suicide," her horrified parents called us. Her husband had reported to the police that she had wanted to kill herself and had asked him to help her. He said he complied by helping her to pull the trigger in a fatal gunshot wound to her head, an absurdity that in some way informed the coroner's conclusion. There was a history of documented abuse in the marriage, including a three-week stay by Amanda in our shelter and two assault charges against her husband, Patrick Smith.

In alliance with Amanda's parents, Judi and Ed Martin, we waged a media campaign that resulted in the coroner's changing his ruling to "undetermined" and Patrick Smith's being tried and convicted of murder. The conviction will never bring back their daughter, but because of our work and that of Judi and Ed, Patrick Smith will serve a lengthy prison system, Amanda's death was not characterized as a "tragic suicide," and the coroner is unlikely to ever again make a ruling of "assisted suicide" on the word of an abusive husband. Following the sentencing, Patrick Smith's defense attorney was quoted by the media as saying, "Some of these victim's groups just have entirely too much power in this community." What better affirmation could we possibly want for our work?

Another example of the sometimes divergent goals of battered-women's programs and the criminal-justice system is demonstrated by the story of Loretta. It has been almost fifteen years since the day I sat at my desk at what was then called the Center for Battered Women. About mid-morning a call came in from a sergeant with the homicide division of the Austin police department. This brave and astute man, someone who had worked murder cases for many years, said, "I have a woman in a holding cell who just shot and killed her husband, called the police, then went and sat on the curb to wait for us to arrive. I have no choice because she has confessed; I have to go through the process. But this woman is no murderer. She didn't see any other options and now she needs your help."

The sergeant told me the woman spoke almost no English and had three children, two sons and a baby daughter. He said the husband told her repeatedly during her pregnancy that if she had a baby girl, he would kill it. He told me the husband was "a really bad guy." The previous night he had held a gun to the baby's head, eventually falling asleep while still holding her with the gun at her head. The terrified mother carefully took the infant away, grasped the gun, and shot and killed her husband. She then woke her two other sleeping children, called the police, and, cradling her sleeping baby, went outside to sit and wait.

My first action was to call a defense attorney, Mack Martinez, who served on our board of directors. He said he would meet me in the lobby of the downtown police station. I then called one of our counselors, a woman named Rosie Guzman who was fluent in both Spanish and English. She was on her way out the door to a family wedding, the cake already boxed and in the back seat of her car, but she said she would meet us at the police station as well. My next call was to Diane McDaniel Rhodes, the shelter director. I told her the story and asked what she thought about the possibility of our bringing a woman into shelter under these circumstances. Diane, always thoughtful and smart said, "It's different, but I think we can make it work."

Within an hour of receiving the call, Mack, Rosie, and I met at the police station. Rosie and Mack talked directly with Loretta, who was still in a holding cell. She was terrified and grieving tremendously over her husband's death, but she never wavered in her story of what had occurred and said that we should do whatever was necessary to her. At least now, she said, her children would be safe. We went next door to the courthouse, where Mack worked magic to have Loretta's case called that afternoon. Miraculously, without yet having served a night in jail, and because of the original intervention of the compassionate sergeant and follow-up by a skilled attorney, she was released by the judge into our custody. Her daughter was still with child protective services, but Loretta and her two sons immediately left with us to stay at the shelter. The baby girl came the next day.

This was by no means the end of the story. Loretta had confessed to murder, and her case was now a part of the system. When the case was referred to the grand jury it was our understanding that the grand jury, given no other choice, voted for indictment but recommended leniency given the circumstances of the case. But once the indictment was handed down, the district attorney's office sought a sentence of life in prison against this young, terrified mother who had taken the only option she had seen to protect her daughter. I doubted that she was in danger of ever again being arrested for anything as offensive as jaywalking. Where could the justice possibly be in separating her from her three young children for life?

We had a good working relationship with the district attorney and his office. These were not lazy, unethical, or unskilled attorneys looking for a quick conviction. We worked with them regularly to assist women and children, but in this case, someone, we believed, had made a bad call. Rather than publicly demand that the charge be changed or withdrawn, we began a careful campaign to inform the district attorney and his office of the extensive support in the community for this woman's case and the unjustness of this particular charge. Had we taken the case to the media and publicly tried to embarrass the district attorney and his staff, we might have won the battle but lost the war, undermining our efforts for other women in the future. Instead, through a letter-writing and phone-calling campaign, we persuaded them to take a second look at the charges they had filed and to rethink their goals.

During this process, Loretta stayed at the shelter with her children, where they all received counseling, and the staff and volunteers worked with her to help her figure out how to support herself and her children going forward.

Our efforts eventually met with success. Loretta received a ten-year sentence, to be served on probation. She would be free to live and work and raise her children unless she reoffended, and then she would serve the balance of her term. Of course, she never reoffended—or even jay-walked—and, perhaps most importantly, she was free to try to give her children a safe and loving home and family.

Of secondary importance were the lessons learned on both sides—by us and by the office of the district attorney and the police department. We learned to support and trust and work with each other in a way we hadn't previously. The outcomes could have been far different, but because of Loretta, the people in the criminal-justice system in Austin and in Travis County learned that they sometimes had to look deeper, beyond the crime, to underlying issues.

I also added the courageous police sergeant to my wall of heroes. He didn't have to make that call—most don't. I later sent him a letter, excerpted below, telling him of the outcome and how his call is what helped to save four lives that day.

I know that as a police officer you don't always know the results of your good works, so I wanted to bring you up to date on this case.

As you may know, we were successful in getting Loretta released from jail and into the shelter, where she stayed for a period of months with her children. We were also able to get her legal counsel and to begin working on her defense. Since leaving the shelter she has continued in weekly support groups at our outreach counseling program, has a full-time job, and takes her two young sons to weekly therapy.

I am most pleased to let you know that Loretta was just sentenced to ten years probation, during which time she will continue in counseling. She was treated with leniency because of the intervention and constant advocacy of the Center for Battered Women and our friends and supporters. We only knew of the circumstances of the case because of a caring and knowledgeable police sergeant who recognized the indicators of a battered woman and made sure that help was made available to her.

Someone recently said that they thought Loretta must have had a "guardian angel sitting on her shoulder." I think you might have been that angel. I wish you could see Loretta and her children today. They are very different from the cowering, frightened people that you took from that home last year. Thank you for caring.

His response back to me was heartfelt — he didn't usually get to see or hear how his actions helped or saved lives. The last I heard, he was still working homicide.

Like the police sergeant, I often lost track of the people in whose lives I had intervened, and I lost track of Loretta after she left the shelter. I knew she was safe, was raising her children, and was living and working in Austin. I also knew that she occasionally continued with counseling but was doing well and didn't see a counselor regularly. One Friday night I was at a traveling carnival set up in a parking lot close to my home. I was there with my children, eating cotton candy, waiting in line for the dizzying rides, and having fun with my family. I noted the group just ahead of me, a mom with her grade-school-age daughter and two adolescent boys, who were clearly enjoying spending an evening together. As their turn approached, the mom, laughing with her kids, turned to me. It was Loretta.

This was the family I had helped to keep together. The three children had been kept from the foster-care system, the mother from incarceration. Our help wasn't merely a temporary fix; we changed four lives and made a difference for Loretta's children — and for their children to come. My eyes meeting Loretta's as she climbed into the seat of the carnival ride is a moment that will forever be imprinted on my memory. I knew then with complete clarity that, yes, I made a difference.

11

lessons
learned from
survivors

The people who have survived and thrived have the ability to hold on to some hope that somewhere inside there still exists a spark of life. Years of abuse and denial of self may hide that spark. It can feel so buried that people forget it exists, especially when it has seemed gone for a very long time. It can be very difficult to access. But given the right circumstances it can still be discovered and then fanned. No matter how a person has been disparaged there is still a human being who holds that internal light, and wherever there is humanity there is hope.

— Sue Snyder, SafePlace counselor
with more than twenty-five years
of experience in the field

A NYONE WHO WORKS IN THE BATTERED-WOMEN'S MOVEMENT knows that we learn more from the survivors than they ever learn from us, the so-called experts and helpers. Battered women are the experts; they help each other learn how to survive. I asked some gifted counselors, case managers, and other service workers what lessons they have learned from survivors. The answers were strikingly similar—they were about trusting, believing, and being a part of a healing community.

The Importance of Being Believed

Melinda Cantu, who began as a social-work intern and is celebrating twenty years at SafePlace this year, currently as the Director of Residential Services, says that "survivors want to know that you understand and do not judge"—that you believe in them. I am reminded that one of the most validating and motivating moments in my personal struggles occurred when the judge said that my ex-husband was a "walking time bomb," and when he went off he would take me with him. Most people think this should have been a frightening moment for me, but it was just the opposite. I already knew the volatility of the situation and the tightrope I walked every day, but I also struggled with being disbelieved and asked what I had done to cause him to hurt me. What I didn't know, until I became involved with the battered-women's movement, is how similar my life was to the lives of hundreds of thousands of other women living with abuse.

"Believing" doesn't mean naïve acceptance, but it does mean offering a place to speak out and to be heard. Other survivors tend to know truth when they hear it spoken. And other survivors are outraged when they hear women make up accusations to gain leverage in child custody or other divorce proceedings. Every time a woman cries wolf to further her own ends, she damages the believability of countless others who are terrified of the risk they take in speaking out. False accusations feed the militant, woman-hating arm of the "father's rights" movement.

Almost every day for more than twenty-five years I have heard women say, "No one believed me…"; "The police didn't believe me when

I said…"; "My family didn't believe…"; "I wasn't believed." I have learned from survivors to "believe."

The Awareness That No One Is Alone

"Survival is a team endeavor; no one has to survive on their own. There are a lot of people on the journey." These are the words of Diane McDaniel Rhodes, who has worked for more than twenty-five years in the field of family violence. Along the way she has been a part of that healing team for thousands of women and children.

I only began to heal once I learned I wasn't alone and started to talk about my abusive marriage with other battered women. We came from different religions, regions of the country, socioeconomic backgrounds, and ethnicities, but we bonded around our common experiences. Battered women help each other to survive and heal. From each other we gain enormous strength and insights. Women can and do survive by going it alone, but it's so much easier to share the journey. This lesson was brought home to many of us on the staff at SafePlace when we were involved with focus groups to determine the design of a new shelter facility. The women told us they wanted a "community." They wanted us to build a space that allowed women to bond in informal settings — around a kitchen table, as they folded laundry, while cooking the day's meal — while still meeting our needs for increased capacity and safety. Survivors told us that creating a sense of community, a space where women could simply talk with each other, was as important to them as feeling safe. We were able to make that happen through a unique shelter design that is described more fully in Chapter 9.

In addition to sharing the journey with other survivors, battered women can and should reach out for assistance from the network of battered-women's programs that crisscross the country. To locate a program in your community call (800) 799-SAFE (7233) or visit the website www.ndvh.org. Volunteers and staff are trained to help callers identify abuse, access services, and advocate for themselves. In the words of a hotline worker, "I talked to a caller today who was looking for information to provide to a survivor who is in a verbally abusive and threatening relationship. I provided the caller with information on accessing our services, and the caller said that she wanted us to know that she appreciates what we do here. She said that she has phoned us several times looking for resources, and that we are always consistent with our work. She said that she has known women who have accessed our shelter, our case-management services, and our counseling services, and she has seen the lives of these women change for the better with our assistance. She said the last person she referred here never thought she could or would make it on her own with her children, but she did. She wanted me to pass on a very heartfelt 'thank you.' She also said, 'One by one, it makes a difference.'"

As I have said previously, getting out of an abusive marriage was the hardest thing I had ever done, and I had friends, a good job, and a supportive family. I would never have been successful had I tried to make it without help.

The Healing Power of Telling One's Story

Wendie Abramson, director of disabilities services at SafePlace, spoke of a man with a cognitive disability who has told her several times how meaningful it is to him to be in a place where he can share his experiences in the hopes that others will take the issue more seriously, where people with disabilities who are abused won't feel so alone with the experience, and where people won't feel pity for him. Wendie says, "Not everyone is in a place where they feel comfortable sharing publicly about such heinous and intrusive experiences, but those who can seem to leap to new highs in their healing process."

By speaking out, Kimberly, whose story is told in Chapter 6, healed some of the shame she carried from her first trial when the defense attorney portrayed her as an invalid whom no one could love. Thomasina, also from Chapter 6, began to understand the ongoing pattern of her sexual, physical, and emotional violation when she began to speak publicly. Her insightful disclosures have helped thousands to better understand the complex relationships between childhood sexual abuse, rape, domestic violence, and economic insecurity.

Perhaps the most important factor in speaking out is that each of us has quit accepting the blame for our abuse, blame that has been assigned by the batterer and often by institutions, our culture, our families, and ourselves.

The Resiliency of Survivors

Survivors are more resilient than I ever thought possible when I first started this work. In Chapter 2 I wrote about meeting the young mothers who were in the shelter in Denver when I started my work there more than twenty-five years ago. I thought the only way they could possibly make it was to find good men to take care of them. I was wrong. These women demonstrated a resiliency beyond anything I expected.

They didn't do it alone; they were lucky enough to connect with services providing housing, child care, and job training. Just as important, they were able to connect with each other. But given the time and the resources, they found the ability and inner strength to overcome enormous obstacles and to build emotionally and economically independent lives for themselves and their children. I have learned never to underestimate humans' resiliency.

The Gift of Fear

More than a decade ago Gavin de Becker wrote an international bestselling book titled *The Gift of Fear*. His book has been published in thirteen languages, appeared on the *New York Times* bestseller list for seventeen weeks, and was profiled on Oprah Winfrey's show. It primarily addresses how to avoid violence outside the family relationship, but much of what he says is also relevant in intimate-partner violence. De Becker urges readers to trust their intuition, their "gift of fear." He talks about patterns associated with violent behavior and he describes preincident indicators. In a chapter titled "Intimate Enemies," de Becker tells us how many women will be murdered over the next twenty-four hours. "In almost every case, the violence that preceded the final violence was a secret kept by several people."[2] He refers to police officers who didn't make arrests, doctors who didn't notify, prosecutors who didn't file charges, and neighbors who ignored the cries from the house next door.

Battered women have internalized and know the "gift of fear." They live in a constant state of heightened awareness, recognize the cycle, and know when they are most in danger. Susan, the woman who came into our shelter eleven times in nine years, learned to recognize the patterns and to know when she needed to seek safety prior to an episode of explosive physical violence. Just as important, everyone working at the shelter learned to trust her instincts, survival instincts that allowed her to live for years in an unstable and dangerous environment until she was able to marshal the resources to leave for good.

Battered women also know intuitively, and sometimes explicitly, that if they upset the status quo by reaching out for help, they put themselves at increased risk. I knew that inviting my mother to help me when I was due to deliver Brandon would put all of us at greater risk. I have learned to trust not only my intuition but also that of other survivors, to believe in and embrace the gift of fear.

The Expertise of Survivors
on Their Own Lives

One of the primary objectives of battered women is to regain the personal power and the control over their lives that have been taken from them. When we designed our new shelter we asked what was important to survivors and listened to what they told us. In almost every instance women wanted the power to make decisions over their lives and the lives of their children. They requested things that most people reading this book take for granted; they wanted to plan their own menus, to cook their own food, to have their own room with their own possessions, to control the temperature in their living space, and to come and go as they pleased. Survivors are the best judges of how to plan their healing and the rest of their lives. As advocates, we are available as guides, educators, champions, and helpers, but ultimately the survivor is in control of charting her own course.

The Ability to Move Beyond Victimization

Most importantly, I learned from other survivors how to heal and move past victimization. Surviving an abusive relationship — enduring all of the difficult times and creating a life free from violence — is hard and never to be minimized. But moving past victimization is something more than surviving; it is healing, knowing that you deserve and are capable of good things.

Not every survivor reaches a point of healing. I have worked with many who totally define themselves through their victimization, women who wait for a white knight to rescue them, or who seem to want to be crowned "Queen for a Day" because of their limitless suffering. These women may have survived abusive marriages, but they are not living the empowered lives that result from true healing.

I learned about healing and empowerment from survivors and from the gifted, compassionate people who have devoted their lives to ending domestic violence. Healing is every bit as difficult as surviving; it is about learning and growing and moving on in a different way. I learned it is possible to become a better you.

building
alliances

We are caught in an inescapable network of mutuality, tied in a single garment of destiny. Whatever affects one directly, affects all indirectly.

— Martin Luther King, Jr.

WHEN LORETTA SHOT HER HUSBAND AND THEN CALLED THE police and waited with her children for them to arrive, the outlook for her future was grim. SafePlace staff and volunteers were able to create opportunities for Loretta because we had spent years building strong alliances with the police department, the criminal court system, and the offices of the district and county attorneys. Building alliances based on feminist values with historically patriarchal organizations is often challenging, but it is central to the work of ending violence against women. Although battered-women's programs are a critical component of the system, they cannot successfully function in a vacuum. It is impossible to talk about battered-women's programs without discussing the partnerships and collaborations that are essential to their success.

Collaboration, which became the buzzword in nonprofit work more than a decade ago, is defined as a mutually beneficial and well-defined relationship entered into by two or more organizations to achieve results they are more likely to accomplish together than alone. When entering into a collaboration, an organization must be willing to embrace complexity and ambiguity; to use the language of "we," "our," and "us"; and to make a commitment of time and resources. Success in building such alliances has been limited, in part because doing so is simply hard work, even when the partnership is between the most well-intentioned organizations with shared goals. In developing collaborations I have decided just to expect conflict, and I have adopted a goal of making that conflict respectful and constructive.

Blending Cultures

Those with whom you begin the collaborative journey may not always be those with whom you end it. When SafePlace began developing its supportive-housing program, our primary collaborative partner was the local Salvation Army. Like SafePlace, the Salvation Army provides shelter and support services for women and children and is dedicated to assisting those with little opportunity; it is usually a choice between receiving support from the Salvation Army or living with your children in your car or under a bridge. In the original agreement SafePlace would build and provide housing, and the Salvation Army would create a child-care program for use by both Salvation Army clients and SafePlace supportive-housing clients.

These two agencies, however, have vastly different organizational cultures; one operates with a feminist-based, egalitarian philosophy, while the other follows a Christian-based, hierarchical, militaristic model. An important but little understood fact about the Salvation Army is that it is a church whose ministry is based on "preaching the gospel of Jesus Christ" while also working to meet human needs. The word "army" is meant to signify that the organization is a fighting force, constantly at war with the powers of evil. It uses military terms; the corps building is sometimes known as the "citadel," the pastor serves as an "officer," and members are "soldiers." Instead of joining the Salvation Army, members are "enrolled" after signing "Articles of War." Through its mission the Salvation Army has done, and continues to do, enormous good in Austin and around the world, but clearly its basic operating premise couldn't be more different from the typical battered-women's program, which grew out of the civil rights movement and is built on a vision of peace for all. In addition, unlike most community-based nonprofits, the Salvation Army doesn't operate with a local governing board of directors. Rather, a centralized board of directors oversees vast regions of the country, and a local advisory board assists in raising funds and connecting the unit to the community.

Our original collaboration was developed with the major who was in charge of the Central Texas Salvation Army. During this development phase I had no idea of the Salvation Army's governance structure and didn't realize the importance of ensuring commitment to our agreement beyond the good will of the major. By the time the HUD grant was secured and operationalized, local leadership had changed and the new major was committed to service in other areas. The two agencies had worked hard at developing open and respectful communication, and there was, and is, enormous good will between them. We were therefore able to constructively discuss the change in direction and develop alternative paths for moving forward. Although the nature and scope of our collaboration was altered, and the Salvation Army didn't provide the child-care component as originally planned, the partnership was a success in that the original goals continued to be met because of our mutual commitment to serving the community, and because of our ability to communicate openly.

It is imperative that members of a collaborative group operate with a shared understanding and respect for each other — for how the respective organizations operate, their cultural norms and values, their limitations, and their expectations. Everyone at the table must be willing to compromise and recognize differences as well as common goals. As organizations founded on feminist principles, most battered-women's programs are committed to operating in a nonjudgmental and inclusive way. However, they can sometimes be rigid and unbending in their very belief in their own openness. In their efforts to be inclusive, they sometimes create difficult environments for organizations and agencies that operate with deeply held religious or hierarchical beliefs. As we found in our collaboration with the Salvation Army, it is imperative that agencies participating in an alliance find their points of intersection and commonality.

An early, and less-than-successful, collaboration also taught me that some things are nonnegotiable. When we were involved in a multiagency effort to provide permanent housing for clients who were leaving shelter, we discovered that the case manager, who worked in our agency but was employed by a partner agency, was making her recommendations to clients by way of tarot card readings. We spoke with the executive director of the partner agency and were told that it wasn't our business how the case manager conducted her work; he was keeping her as a case manager, and she would continue to work with our clients. He further stated that we were "nothing but a bunch of red-headed lesbians from Fort Worth." (There is no sense in even trying to explain that statement.) We chose to discontinue our participation with that agency rather than have our clients' lives guided through tarot card readings.

This collaboration plainly didn't work. It is a bit of an understatement to say that the two organizations lacked a respectful working relationship, trust, and mutually agreed upon goals, outcomes, and work styles.

Elsewhere in the book I've touched on the importance of building alliances between battered-women's programs and criminal-justice agencies. These collaborations can often be difficult. Battered-women's advocates may balk at the hierarchical, militaristic, top-down structure predominant in law enforcement. In addition, every battered-women's advocate has worked with more than one woman who has been victimized by a husband or boyfriend in law enforcement. When an officer of the law abuses not only his partner but also the power of his position, it fosters a sense of mistrust between battered-women's advocates and police officers. However, law enforcement officials and battered-women's programs are also deeply aware of the necessity of working together. Advocates want the police to respond quickly and appropriately when they are called, and members of law enforcement value having a shelter available to house women and children in need. They recognize better than most that they are unable to fully protect some women. Given a shared vision, and concrete goals and objectives, in most instances both sides work hard at figuring out methods for bridging their differences.

For those of us who have worked for many years in family violence, it is amazing to look back and see the phenomenal changes that have occurred over the past thirty years in the relationship between law enforcement and domestic-violence organizations. In Austin, for example, we have replaced suspicion with open conversation. As recently as twelve years ago, SafePlace staff grumbled when police officers came to the shelter and were hesitant to allow them in for fear of how shelter residents might feel. A couple of years later, when we were building the new shelter facility and considering whether or not to remain a confidential location, we chose to actively engage law enforcement agencies in helping us to make that decision and in ensuring safety for the residents. In a surprising turnaround, we ended up hiring off-duty, uniformed officers to provide security at the shelter.

Informal Alliances

A true collaboration, which involves the sharing of goals, resources, and time, can be expensive and difficult to operate. Yet collaborations are frequently touted as the best way to provide service. While I agree that they can be effective, there are times when alternative strategies are equally vital. Cooperation and cross-referral are frequently just as effective as formal collaborations or contracts. Family violence shelters in Texas work in this cooperative manner without memorandums of understanding or letters of agreement in place. There is common agreement among Texas shelters that they exist as a network to serve battered women in the state. If one is full, then a neighboring shelter is called; if it is too dangerous for a battered woman to stay in the town where she lives, a shelter in another town, or sometimes even in another state, is called. It is a remarkable, unspoken agreement between organizations. There are no legal contracts, payments, or invoicing for services rendered, or quid-pro-quo expectations. Witnessing this level of cooperation is a heartening part of working with battered women.

Cooperation between shelters also occurs nationwide. Many times clients are moved across states lines because of particular safety concerns, proximity to family and job opportunities, or a program's specialized focus in some area of service. Several years ago SafePlace received a request from a shelter in a major city in a neighboring state asking us to admit Fatima, an older woman with a severe mental illness who was being persecuted by her conservative Muslim family because she had been raped. Fatima's family blamed her for the assault, and they were so ashamed of her they had a contract placed on her life. The shelter workers knew she was not safe in her city because of the family's far-reaching wealth, prestige, and influence, and that she must be moved to another city where the family couldn't find her. They contacted Austin's SafePlace because it has a national reputation for expertise in sheltering people with disabilities; the staff quite literally wrote the book on serving people with the dual issues of mental illness and victimization (*Beyond Labels: Working with Abuse Survivors with Mental Illness Symptoms or Substance Abuse Issues*). SafePlace also has a reputation for being open, flexible, and accommodating in unusual circumstances; it doesn't restrict admission solely to those experiencing violence in intimate-partner relationships. Fatima was accepted into the SafePlace shelter, and she has since moved on to be moderately independent and safe, away from her family.

Working Together to Change
and Improve the System

Even when a particular agency is deemed most efficient and effective in providing a particular service, shelter being a good example, seldom is it adequate for any agency to work without assistance from other community partners. In Austin, as in most major cities, there are a plethora of task forces, coalitions, and planning bodies that work together. The alphabet soup of these groups is, at first blush, overwhelming. They include the Victim Services Task Force (VSTF), the Sexual Assault Response Team (SART), and the Family Violence Task Force (FVTF), all of which exist for different but related purposes: to improve the lives of, and the official response to, victims of sexual and family violence and other types of abuse.

SafePlace commits significant time and energy to participating in and leading these groups. There have been many occasions when, as executive director of SafePlace, I would question how on earth we could afford to be at each meeting. But I ended up believing that it is frequently through these groups, and in partnership with others, that we are able to achieve the improvements in the system and the social change that we seek. Each of the task forces amplifies the voices of the involved individuals in order to advocate, educate, and ensure that the systems work for a victim, instead of revictimizing her. When Kimberly Wisseman went to court to file charges against her abuser, she was not believed, and justice was not served. Our hope is that today, should someone with similar circumstances seek justice in Austin, her or his experience would be different because of the work we have done with other agencies that also have a responsibility to protect.

In Austin, SafePlace worked with other groups to develop a specialized domestic-violence court, led by longtime judge Mike Denton. Judge Denton has learned about the dynamics of family violence and brings that understanding to his work. When I think about Kimberly's experience I know without a doubt that had her case been heard in front of Judge Denton the outcome would have been different. This humble man has not only educated himself on women's issues, family violence, and sexual abuse, but he also went so far as to complete the forty-hour volunteer training offered by the former Austin Rape Crisis center (now Safe-Place). He tells about going to the hospital to learn about SANE (Sexual Assault Nurse Examiner) forensic exams. He was the only man in the training who was willing to climb up on the exam table and put his feet in the stirrups, and he says it was life-changing to experience a portion of the vulnerability and exposure a woman feels in that position.

Along with Judge Denton, the Travis County attorney's office trains other criminal-justice officials nationwide in how to create a specialized court comprised of personnel with in-depth knowledge of family violence. If you were to ask Judge Denton why the court was developed, he would give credit to SafePlace and the Family Violence Task Force, and to the gentle, "honeylike" advocacy that was used to impress upon the powers-that-be the need for this specialized court. Judge Denton has set aside a special room off his courtroom where victims and their volunteer advocates can meet, wait, and prepare to go to court. He is yet another of the unsung heroes who quietly and courageously go about their work, changing and saving lives every day.

Effective Partnering to Assist the Needy

One of the most efficient collaborations I have seen got its start when a group of nonprofit executive directors had lunch together to share their frustration that their clients were unable to engage in their services because the clients' financial needs always took precedence. These services were usually dedicated to moving clients toward greater self-sufficiency and economic empowerment, but the clients couldn't seem to get off the treadmill long enough to work for the future.

That first, informal meeting eventually resulted in local government and nonprofit leaders coming together from across various disciplines, agencies, and focus areas: domestic violence, AIDS, children's health, disability services, elder services, and the working poor. All agreed that the current system for distributing financial assistance was inadequate, and until it was improved each agency, and the clients it served, faced serious barriers. To test this assumption, the group followed one woman through the system to see what really happened to her when she sought help.

Mary, a formerly battered woman and the single parent of two young children, lived on the edge of poverty and needed emergency assistance. She had a full-time job that paid $8.50 an hour. If she didn't work, she didn't get paid. When the choice was between missing work to attend a parent–teacher conference or buying groceries, she risked being labeled an uninterested or inadequate parent by the school. Mary received a partial subsidy for child care, used the bus with her two children for transportation, and had some family support, but not much. Her ex-husband paid child support erratically. In addition, one of her children had a chronic health condition. She missed almost three weeks of work when he was too ill to go to school, and she started looking for financial assistance when she faced eviction because she wasn't able to pay her $600 a month rent.

Mary sought help from eleven different sources: a governmental agency, two nonprofits, four churches, and friends and family. She received some type of financial assistance from the governmental agency, one nonprofit, three churches, and a family member. In order to receive assistance from all these helpers, Mary had to tell her story numerous times, fill out multiple intake forms, and take four partial days off work for appointments. Ultimately, she secured $450 a month in assistance, not enough money to make her rent payment. She also ended up losing even more money from missed work, which caused the problem to continue into the following month. The system simply did not work for Mary, and it doesn't work for others living on the edge of poverty. Mary lives in Austin, Texas, but her story is repeated hundreds of thousands of times in numerous cities across the nation. It is often even worse in rural communities with no public transportation and located many miles between services, or in other large cities like Chicago, where services are even more disconnected than in smaller cities like Austin.

From Mary's plight, and the experiences of others like her, sprang the idea for the creation of the Best Single Source project (BSS). A person seeking assistance goes to only one agency, the one that is best suited to address the person's problem. For instance, victims of family violence are referred to SafePlace. Instead of referring her to other organizations for financial aid, something that happens in many communities, SafePlace draws on a central repository of funds that are available to all BSS partner agencies. Each partner agency can grant financial assistance of up to $1,500 per family. The client is required to agree to work with a case manager for at least three months to address the underlying or causative issue.

There are currently nine partners in the BSS collaboration who share a centralized database and the responsibility of raising money for the project. In the six years since the program's inception, thousands of people have been assisted, and well over 80 percent never have to come back for more financial assistance. This arrangement is respectful to clients because they do not have to repeat their stories to multiple helpers; it is efficient because clients do not have to seek help from multiple sources, a task that is time-consuming and expensive; it is effective because it solves clients' immediate financial problem; and it is successful because it helps them to address the real causes of their poverty. Obviously this program is not for everybody, and people suffering from chronic or lifelong poverty may not benefit, but for many it has offered a solution to dire financial hardships.

As one of the founding partner agencies, SafePlace has been thrilled to be part of a project that not only helps individuals but also improves a system that was grossly inadequate. However, not everyone has understood why domestic-violence workers would spend so much time on a collaboration that was not focused on sexual or domestic violence, but rather on poverty. What I have learned with absolute certainty is that Maslow's hierarchy of needs remains a solid framework for considering how best to provide services to a client. A person's most basic needs — food, housing, and clothing — must be met in order for them to think about anything else. I think this is especially true for women with children. Making sure the kids have food on the table and a roof over their heads is generally the most pressing concern of most mothers, followed closely by physical safety.

Providing Organizational Leadership

One of the strengths and one of the weaknesses of the Best Single Source collaboration is the number of partners. Generally speaking, the more partners a collaboration has, the more complex and difficult it can be. In these cases, success or failure often depends on the leadership of the collaboration and of the partner agencies. Sometimes it is not immediately obvious why we need to be leaders. This happened in the early 1990s when we joined the local Homeless Coalition. Board members wondered why I was spending my time attending these meetings and why I encouraged staff at the Center for Battered Women (as SafePlace was then called) to accept time-consuming leadership positions in the coalition. The Homeless Coalition had not always been very effective, had even been divisive and destructive at times, and the Center for Battered Women hadn't participated in any way before then. Staff at the Center for Battered Women historically felt there were more pressing priorities on which they should spend their time, and our lack of participation, because we were operating a major agency that provided services to a significant number of homeless people, hurt our reputation with the homeless-service-provider community. The word in the nonprofit community was that the Center for Battered Women was closed, elitist, and didn't play well with others. And the perception was true; we were inwardly focused at that time in our organizational development.

My goal was to be more involved in the community. We had been successful in forming partnerships with law enforcement, so I knew we could productively work with other agencies, beginning with the Homeless Coalition. SafePlace's strategic plan identified increased shelter capacity and the creation of transitional-housing programs as our highest priorities over the next three to five years. If we were to be successful in securing public funding to create and expand these services, we had to be at the forefront in identifying and addressing the intersection between homelessness and domestic violence.

The simple truth is that battered women living in shelters are homeless. They are the hidden homeless, but they are homeless nevertheless. A 1990 Ford Foundation study found that 50 percent of homeless women and children were fleeing abuse.[1] Another study found that 92 percent of homeless women reported being severely physically or sexually abused at some point in their lives.[2] I have long conjectured how differently the general population might view homelessness if we were to line up all of the homeless women and children and parade them down Main Street America.

After our agency had been involved for a couple of years with the Homeless Coalition, the Travis County plan was altered to more comprehensively address not only the needs of the homeless men who panhandled on corners and lined up at night for beds at a homeless shelter, but also those of the many invisible homeless families — the majority consisting of women and children made homeless because their own homes weren't safe. Following the adoption of this plan, the Center for Battered Women was prepared to apply for and receive HUD funds for transitional housing.

Through participation in the Homeless Coalition, SafePlace also became partners in a successful multiagency alliance called Passages. The Passages program helps individuals leave homelessness through the use of community-housing options. Were it not for active participation in the Homeless Coalition, SafePlace and the other Passages partners could not have been as successful in addressing the complex needs of homelessness.

Keeping collaborations alive requires being able to share power and reach compromise. Communication is a key element in a successful alliance. Nonprofit managers are exceptionally good at collaborations because they know that almost all nonprofits succeed or fail based on the ability to build, maintain, and grow relationships. My opinion is that organizations dealing with sexual and domestic violence, as experts in healthy relationships, should also be expert collaborators.

Partnering with School Districts

A groundbreaking partnership for SafePlace has been with the Austin Independent School District (AISD). As with most collaborations, this one had an interesting beginning. In the 1980s a high-school counselor phoned the Center for Battered Women because she had witnessed a student being abused by her boyfriend. The counselor said that she had been learning about domestic violence and that the shoving, berating, and yelling looked a lot like wife abuse, except in this case the students were young and not married. The counselor asked if someone from the center could come to the school and speak with the female student. At that moment, SafePlace's groundbreaking program Expect Respect was born.

What has sustained this program is its organic growth. It was started not by the agency or AISD administrators but by school counselors who were closest to the students and who recognized and responded to a problem. It grew primarily through word of mouth. School counselors told their peers at other schools that staff from the Center for Battered Women had helped their kids. More and more counselors called and asked agency staff to come to their campus and talk to students they were worried about. Eventually the counselors encouraged their principals to formalize the relationship. Throughout the history of Expect Respect, school counselors have been the biggest advocates, greatest collaborators, and best friends to agency staff and students alike.

Years later, after our agency had worked with well over a dozen campuses in AISD, we entered into a formal agreement with the district. The Austin Independent School District has been supporting the Expect Respect program for over two decades, first as a partner and collaborator, and later in a formal funding relationship. The unique partnership has enabled SafePlace to develop a comprehensive dating-violence program that engages *all* members of the school community: students, counselors, teachers, cafeteria workers, parents, school administrators, and others.

Sadly, a tragedy resulted in a strengthening of the relationship. Ortralla Mosley, a fifteen-year-old cheerleader and dance-squad leader at Reagan High School was murdered in the school hallway by her former boyfriend, Marcus McTear, a popular sixteen-year-old football player. Ortralla and her friends had gone to school officials asking for help because she was afraid of McTear. They told her to leave the school. As she hid in the hallways, trying to leave, Marcus found her and stabbed her six times, including through her heart and through her skull, piercing her brain.

Ortralla's mother, Carolyn Mosley Samuels, said that after Ortralla became a cheerleader, McTear grew more possessive and domineering and complained about the kinds of clothes Ortralla wore, insisting they were too revealing. When Ortralla was getting ready to break up with him, he tried to slash his own throat. After Ortralla's death, McTear's violence in earlier relationships came to light. He had abused one young woman so badly that she changed schools and was, at the time of Ortralla's death, involved in the SafePlace Expect Respect program at her new school. Her mother later told the media that her daughter came home crying after arguments with McTear. When she showed up one day with bruises, the mother called the school principal to ask for assistance and protection for her daughter, but she received no response. McTear eventually pushed the young woman down a flight of stairs. Her mother, increasingly terrified for her daughter's life, took action to move her to another school.

In 2003 McTear was sentenced in the Texas Juvenile Justice System to forty years behind bars. When he turned twenty-one, he was transferred into an adult penitentiary where he remains today.

In response to Ortralla's tragic murder, AISD, with help from Safe-Place, developed a district-wide teen-dating violence policy. During the 2007 Texas legislative session, Representative Dawnna Dukes, a graduate of Reagan High School, introduced a bill requiring that all school districts in the state have a teen-dating violence policy. It was passed into law. One of the leading proponents for passage of the bill was Carolyn Mosley Samuels, Ortralla's mother. SafePlace staff and board members, along with partners from AISD, also testified for passage of the legislation based on the belief that all members of the school community—

faculty, staff, students, and parents—play important roles in preventing dating violence and promoting healthy relationship behaviors. The bill states, "Dating violence includes the use of physical, sexual, verbal, or emotional abuse by a person to harm, threaten, intimidate, or control another person in a relationship of a romantic or intimate nature, regardless of whether that relationship is continuing or has concluded."

AISD now funds the Expect Respect program, though SafePlace continues to raise and invest significant resources to provide the services. SafePlace recently hired a young woman named Joli to work in the Expect Respect program at Reagan High School. Joli had been one of Ortralla Mosley's best friends and knows firsthand how it feels to fear for a friend, to ask for help for her, and to see it denied. Joli is also a member of the Public Offenders, a hip-hop band that produces socially conscious music, much of it about ending violence. A song about Ortralla is featured on the Public Offenders' CD, *Dropping Jewels*. Joli, age twenty-two, uses her fabulous voice and her personal experience to help youth from her neighborhood and school by bringing awareness to the issue of dating violence in a way that kids can hear.

As the experience with AISD shows, effective nonprofit agencies are integrated into their communities and try to respond when a new need is highlighted. They also know what services other community agencies provide and avoid duplicating them. In the spirit of cooperation, they set aside ego, turfs, and worries about funding to achieve a greater good.

In the best-case scenario, a project, agency, or collaboration ends when the problem is solved. In reality, however, more often than not it ends due to a loss of funding. The Passages project, a dynamic and successful program, is dwindling down, and will likely not continue. HUD, the lead funder, has shifted its priorities, and new homeless programs are positioning themselves to receive the governmental funds that have flowed to Passages for many years. Passages has been tremendously successful in achieving the goal of ending homelessness for the families that have participated in the program, but the problem of homelessness has endured, and new ideas and programs are vying to step to the forefront.

Collaborations are challenging, time-consuming, and expensive; participating in them comes at a great cost to any organization. At the same time, successful collaborations are unmatched in making enormous change. The African proverb "it takes a village to raise a child" can be applied to the remarkable transformation that a group of organizations can achieve when they work together toward common goals of service, change, and improvement.

13

lessons learned through leading domestic-violence programs

If you're going to go for the long jump, you're bound to get a little sand in your shorts.

— Anonymous

A NYONE WHO HAS WORKED WITH ME WILL BE QUICK TO TELL you that I am most assuredly not a counselor. I have spent years working with and around counselors, social workers, and other social-service professionals, but my gift is not in helping people on their personal journeys. I have two modes: "Let me fix it for you," and "Buck up, princess," neither of which is a particularly useful way to empower someone to help herself and to find her own way. My strength lies in figuring out how to grow and lead organizations. I have been an executive director of private, nonprofit, community-based, human-service agencies for over twenty-five years—a long time by anyone's standards. As an executive director I have worked for numerous volunteer boards of directors and struggled to raise millions of dollars to support and grow the agencies for which I've been responsible. Much of what I've learned is essential to the care, feeding, management, and growth of any nonprofit, but particularly for battered-women's programs.

I took over the reins at Safehouse for Battered Women, in Denver, Colorado, at a point when the agency had been closed down because of mismanagement. When we conducted the previous year's financial audit the cancelled checks were in a box under a former board treasurer's bed. I remember many sleepless nights trying to figure out how I could make the next payroll by holding back my own paycheck, or by telling United Way that I would pick up their check in person rather than waiting for it to arrive in the mail, or by delaying payment of bills until the latest possible date I could do so without incurring a penalty. I often had to utilize all three strategies simultaneously.

All of this is to say that running a nonprofit is not for the faint of heart; it is really hard work. And running a program for battered women is, I believe, truly only for those who have made it their personal mission.

I credit the success of the agencies I have led to several factors, not the least of which has been my likely good fortune, as opposed to my good sense, at having taken the helm of organizations that had vital and focused missions, and that were operating in the right place at the right time. Despite this good luck, I have learned some important lessons along the way, lessons that I will take this opportunity to share. I would love to say that when it comes to learning from these lessons I have uniformly followed my own advice, but, of course, that wouldn't be the truth. Mostly, I have learned through my mistakes, and sometimes I have made similar mistakes more than once.

Stay Focused on the Mission

Any nonprofit agency should maintain an almost obsessive focus on its mission, a task that is sometimes easier said than done. When the mission expands or changes, as happened when the Center for Battered Women merged with the Austin Rape Crisis Center to become SafePlace, the shift should be thoughtful and planned, rather than resulting from "mission creep," which often happens when organizations chase scarce dollars, or at the whim of the leadership.

SafePlace went through an extensive process to be able to apply for low-income-housing tax credits as part of our plan to build an affordable-housing apartment community. Several members of the board of directors correctly asked, "Is creating permanent housing really a part of our mission?" The question prompted us to put together a task force made up of representatives from the board, staff, and clients. They were assigned the job of comprehensively analyzing the issue of affordable housing as it related to battered women, the need in our community, SafePlace's capacity to provide the service, alternative housing providers, and what SafePlace's role should be.

Giving clients a voice as a part of the task force was critically important. Board members listened to Thomasina, the former shelter and supportive-housing client who, despite the advantages of a graduate degree and numerous interventions, had very nearly ended up homeless with her daughters. She spoke with piercing honesty and eloquence about her struggles to find and maintain safe and affordable housing for herself and her girls. As she spoke, the board members who had questioned Safe-Place's role in providing permanent housing began to better understand the intersection between domestic violence and the need for affordable housing. Thomasina's story, and those of other clients, were more important in the decision-making process than all the research, data, and statistics provided by staff. This illustrates a second, equally important lesson.

Remain Customer Driven

Being a customer-driven organization has helped SafePlace many times to maintain its focus on its mission. The insights and opinions of current and former clients are valued and are incorporated into the operations and governance of the agency.

When I started as executive director at Safehouse for Battered Women, in Denver, I didn't tell anyone I had been a battered woman. I thought that if people knew, they wouldn't trust my judgment to lead the agency. In the years since, I have made a 180-degree turn. I now believe that my perspective as a formerly battered woman is valuable and should be included in planning and implementing services. Not to do so further promulgates the patriarchal system that deems women unable to fully participate in decision-making about their own lives and bodies.

Customers should be defined as more than just clients, depending on the activity or service provided. Donors should be regularly involved in discussions about fund-raising and should be called on to expand and lead resource-development activities. Engaging staff in discussions relevant to their lives and work is also essential. Who better to ask about preferences for employee benefits than the employees who will be most impacted by the decision? When given a specific problem and the parameters associated with possible solutions, the staff, as the customers in that scenario, should be engaged in deciding on solutions.

Clients, as customers, should be an integral part of the problem-solving process associated with most major decisions. At SafePlace we've involved clients and former clients in several ways. Clients were consulted when we designed the new shelter and when we were making the decision about no longer maintaining a confidential location. And we've recruited significant numbers of staff, volunteers, and board members from the rosters of our former clients.

Keep the Board Leadership Engaged

During my first ten years as an executive director I continually questioned why anyone would have thought that a volunteer board of directors could possibly be an effective form of governance. How could a disparate group of people, ill-informed about the work of the organization but given total power over its future, be the best method for maintaining an agency's continuity and success? In my second decade as a nonprofit executive I came to realize that an effective and informed board of directors is, in fact, the most important tool for success any nonprofit organization can have. My most important job as CEO is to make certain this diverse group is well-informed and appropriately engaged so that when important decisions must be made the board is prepared to step up and do so.

A primary reason for the success of SafePlace has been the engagement and involvement of its board of directors. In the early days the members of the board were directly responsible for the day-to-day operations of the agency—volunteering on overnight shifts, taking the sheets and towels home to wash them, and writing the grants that funded the agency's meager budget. As the organization grew, the board's focus shifted to that of a more mature agency. Professional accountants were hired to manage the financial reporting; licensed master's-level social workers, many of whom are regionally and nationally recognized as leaders in the field, were hired to work in and develop programs; grant writers, attorneys, and various other professionals stepped in to take over many of the operational tasks that had originally consumed the board's time. The board was then free to focus its attention on governance, policy, and—always—fund-raising.

Every person who agrees to serve on a nonprofit board of directors should agree to assist with fund-raising. That assistance can take many different forms, but every director should commit first and foremost to making the agency a priority for their personal philanthropy and to making a "stretch" gift. Many organizations set specific dollar amounts that each board member must give or obtain through fund-raising. I am not a big supporter of this approach. I have found that individuals too often consider the dictated amount a "ceiling" for their donation rather than a "floor," believing they have already met their commitment. In addition, if diversity is an important consideration for the board of directors, as it should be for every domestic-violence program, a "give-get" policy can be a disincentive to joining for potential board members of limited means and without access to people of affluence.

By clearly stating the expectation up front that resource development is a critically important part of board service, and then motivating directors to care about and support the organization, I have seen boards step up and give or raise millions of dollars. When they are invested in the work and mission of the agency, recognize a compelling need, and have committed to the hard work of raising money, the board can be the best fund-raising tool an organization has.

Thomasina became a member of the SafePlace board of directors at a time when she was actively struggling to avoid homelessness; making financial contributions was clearly not a consideration for her. But she was able to tell her story and to influence others to give. Her generosity of spirit was instrumental in helping us to raise millions of dollars, and, as important, her keen insights and participation on the board consistently assisted in steering board decisions. Conversely, Donna Stockton-Hicks, the sexual abuse survivor and formerly battered woman whose story is also told in Chapter 6, was able to bring her knowledge, her personal story, *and* millions of dollars in contributions. Both women's participation was critical and important to the work of the board and the future of the organization.

A board of directors is also tasked with employing the agency's chief executive — meaning they are responsible for hiring and firing the executive director. This is one of the most important, if not *the* most important, jobs entrusted to a board, and it is one I have seen seemingly smart and savvy boards fail miserably at, particularly when it comes to the continued employment of founder/leaders. All too often, the community and the board regard a nonprofit agency as "belonging" to a founder/leader, the person who had the original vision and concept. But organizations are given nonprofit, tax-exempt status because they agree to provide a service to their community. The moment this tax-exempt status is accepted, the founder/leader forsakes her or his personal ownership of the idea, and the organization and ownership is transferred to the community, with a board of directors that holds it in trust.

A board will never be as informed and educated as staff members think they should be. A board should be a diverse group if they are charged with representing the community the organization serves. The strength, commitment, and involvement of the board of directors is probably the most important determination of whether an agency will stay alive and prosper. A nonprofit organization belongs to the community it serves — not to the staff, or the CEO, or even the board of directors. However, the board does, I repeat, hold the organization in trust for the community.

Recruit the Right Team

Rarely am I the smartest person in the room, but I am almost always able to tell you who is — a talent that has stood me in good stead throughout my career. Recognizing and recruiting the right team at every level is essential to the success of any organization. Hire carefully, have an expectation of excellence, and cut your losses early if you see it isn't working.

I once ran for office, and I was quick to tell the people who recruited me, "There are a number of people in this community who don't particularly like me because there are a number of people whom I have fired." I learned to cut my losses early. If you think it won't work out, it almost never does.

Most managers spend 75 percent of their time trying to manage the least productive workers in their companies. I know that I am certainly as guilty as the next person of spending too much of my time working with the employee who is unproductive, is passive-aggressive, undermines the team and the mission, and constantly produces late and sloppy work. I think women are guiltier of this than men. We see it as our role to be the nurturer, to help people succeed, and to be the caregiver. This is a particular problem with battered-women's and other violence-prevention programs. Although customers and former clients provide an important voice to have in the mix, sometimes these are individuals who haven't worked through their own victimization and still see the world in terms of oppressor and oppressed.

I firmly believe that our role as caregivers should not be confused with our role as managers. They are different. And we do no one any favors by carrying bad employees — not the underperformer and not her coworkers.

I had an employee at the Denver Safehouse whom I relied on heavily. She had all of the right credentials and had been with the agency for a very long time. We had experienced a lot of staff turnover, and it was my impression that the staff who remained were intensely loyal to her. I also knew that she was an active alcoholic and that it was possible her drinking was affecting her work. When finally forced to confront the situation I was terrified of the repercussions. Would she quit and take most of the staff with her? How would this affect my reputation in the service-provider community? After all, I was just a formerly battered woman who was in over her head — or so I had been led to believe by this staff member. When I offered her the option of either time off for treatment to control her drinking, or to be let go, she chose to be fired. To my amazement, the next day the rest of the staff sent me flowers. They had been as cowed into submission as I had, and their gratefulness at my finally taking action has stayed with me to this day.

I believe it is important to recruit and hire based on qualities and values; these are often more important than a person's specific background or expertise. I would rather hire a director of development who is passionate about the mission of the organization *and* has the necessary qualities to be successful in fund-raising — is organized, is a good writer, is a skilled verbal communicator, works well with a team, is a good listener, and builds effective relationships with others — than someone who merely has a lot of experience in fund-raising. A person can learn how to be a great fund-raiser, but it is impossible to teach passion for the mission.

All employees and volunteers should also embrace the core values that drive the organization. That doesn't mean that everyone should be the same—definitely not. Recruit for diversity of ethnicity, sexuality, age, and whatever other issues are important to the work, but an employer or stakeholder won't be successful if staff and volunteers fail to embrace the core values that drive the organization. At Chicago Foundation for Women, the organization I took over in January 2009, the core values are equality, empowerment, diversity, collaboration, and integrity. All staff, board members, volunteers, and grantee organizations have also committed to these values and work toward developing effective ways of measuring progress toward achieving goals that are linked both to these values and to specific service activities the foundation participates in.

A very wise man once told me, "If you are spending your time looking over your shoulder and covering your backside, you can't have vision." In other words, recruit the right team and then get out of their way.

Manage for the Best Among Us Rather than the Worst Among Us

Once you get the right team, then you need to empower them to do their jobs. I learned one of my most important management lessons over twenty years ago when I ran the Developmental Preschool and Daycare, in Laramie, Wyoming. Trying to harness the power and energy of more than a hundred preschoolers is a trying task at best. Every time we turned around some child was doing something new that made us want to tear our hair out, so we promptly created a new rule to address it. Eventually we had so many rules and policies that the staff couldn't keep track of them, let alone the kids. Finally, a special-education teacher sat us all down and said, "This is crazy. Let's figure out what is really important."

I don't remember exactly what we came up with, but I do know we asked ourselves, "What are the fundamental guidelines that should steer everything else?" One was about not posing a danger to others, or hurting them. A second was about not posing a danger to or hurting yourself. Once we had our basic guidelines we viewed all situations through the lens of those rules and everything became much clearer. No more trying to figure out what particular infraction had been broken. Most important, our guidelines were made clear to staff and parents, and everyone began to learn and use judgment instead of just trying to remember a plethora of rules and restrictions. And don't all of us want nothing more for our children than for them to learn to use good judgment? How better to learn it than to see it modeled by the adults in their lives?

This lesson stood me in good stead as I took over the increasingly complex business of running battered-women's and rape-crisis programs. There is simply no way that we can create a rule for every eventuality that might arise in these programs that deal with real-life drama and tragedies. Staff and volunteers have to feel empowered and educated to make decisions in complex situations for which there are no clear-cut playbooks.

There also has to be room to sometimes make the wrong decision and then to use it as a learning experience. If an employee is repeatedly making the wrong decision, then they may not be in the right place. I look for patterns. Do people use good judgment, make decisions, and then move on, having learned the lessons from those decisions, both good and bad? When a shelter employee made a disastrous mistake that resulted in a young girl being sexually molested by another child on our premises, the employee wasn't let go, or punished, or even admonished. She saw her mistake, learned from it, and put in place additional measures and strategies to make sure it would never happen again.

That employee was, and is to this day, one of the best among us — and worthy of time, attention, and support. And she manages those around her in the same way, particularly in all of her interactions with clients. We should aim to create environments where we learn from our mistakes and move on. Creating a rigid environment in which there is no room for mistakes is antithetical to the philosophy of the battered-women's movement and fails to foster innovation and learning.

Attend to the Business of the Agency

Too often nonprofits seem to forget the "Incorporated" part of their name. They fail to tend to the business side of their operations. It is wonderful to feel good and to do good work, but if the work is to continue, then nonprofit agencies must also attend to the grant reporting, bookkeeping, database management, human resources, and myriad other details that make up the business of doing business. The service needs can be so overwhelmingly intense and huge that any resources directed toward building and maintaining management systems and infrastructure can feel directly competitive with helping just one more family. However, if infrastructure and management systems aren't attended to, the agency risks losing the ability to continue its work.

In my early years at SafePlace I would do a nominal group process each year with the staff. (This was before the employee roster grew so large that any type of group process became unwieldy.) A nominal group process is a highly structured exercise designed to ensure that each member of a group has equal opportunity to engage in meeting an agreed-upon goal. As you would expect, the most important objectives identified by the staff always involved increasing the availability of services for clients. The staff-on-the-ground are usually the ones who know best where the gaps and needs exist in the areas of service provision. However, one particular year I was in for a huge surprise. We had just begun the tremendous growth phase that would eventually result in SafePlace becoming one of the largest organizations of its kind, and we were struggling with that growth. I ended up calling it "the toilet paper year."

Once everyone was heard from, votes had been tallied and weighted for priority, and varied but similar thoughts had been compiled and organized, we determined that the most important issue for the SafePlace staff wasn't creating more shelter beds, or adding another children's counselor, or recruiting more volunteers to answer the hotline—it was infrastructure. In the discussions involving infrastructure I heard repeatedly what it was like to lack sufficient technology to do one's job: to have outdated phone systems, insufficient office supplies, convoluted systems for data collection, and—yes—not enough toilet paper! Think about it: In a large organization that is 95 percent staffed by women, and in which almost all of the clients are women and girls, toilet paper should not be a luxury. You men reading this may not immediately understand, but women everywhere will get it.

That was the year we all said, "Oops, it's time to focus inwardly for a bit. Let's try to get our house in order and make sure things work before we enter this next big growth phase." Had we not spent that year focusing on things like data collection, bookkeeping, supply chain, human-resources management, and technology, I am convinced we would have failed miserably when it came time to make the next big leap in our organizational growth.

The value of some of the systems we created weren't immediately apparent to me. The development team hounded me to provide them with all the information I held in my head about the convoluted relationships and history with major donors. I balked at having to spend this time, but they just kept coaxing the information from me. When I left SafePlace and took over the helm at the Chicago Foundation for Women I had a lightbulb moment when I discovered by looking at the foundation's donor files that various people through the years had meticulously updated notes and contacts for all major donors. Had they not done so I would have come in operating blind. I said to myself, "So this is what SafePlace's development staff was trying so hard to get out of me!"

Creating an infrastructure that can sustain a growing organization has always been, and continues to be, a difficult task. One of the most challenging, but important, parts of the job is to develop systems that can support the agency while allowing it to be nimble and responsive. Sometimes, however, the business side of the agency may take over all aspects of the organization—the mission becomes subjugated to the day-to-day operations.

Many business executives are disdainful of nonprofit management, thinking all a nonprofit needs to be successful is the rigor of a good business model. They see it as a kind of laid-back retirement farm. However, most former for-profit executives who have successfully made the transition to a nonprofit career will tell you that it's actually harder to succeed in the nonprofit world than in the for-profit world because the goals are more complex and intangible. A for-profit corporation measures its success by increasing shareholder or ownership value—by making money—

whereas a nonprofit's goals tend to be behavioral, which are much harder to measure. In Jim Collins's monograph *Good to Great and the Social Sector*, he points out, "In business, money is both an input (a resource for achieving greatness) and an output (a measure of greatness). In the social sectors, money is only an input, and not a measure of greatness."[1] Management in the nonprofit sector is also complicated by the fact that the CEOs almost always have less authority and control than their for-profit counterparts, because they answer to a much wider range of stake-holders. Finally, compared to the corporate world, the nonprofit sector is underfunded, understaffed, underresourced, and undertrained.

The infrastructure and the management systems of a nonprofit are in place to support the mission and the work of the organization. Those systems must allow the agency to be responsive and accountable to the community it serves. Again, never, ever lose sight of the mission—and tending to the business details of the operation is crucial to allowing you to do that.

Work Toward a Vision for the Future

In every job, I have been labeled a visionary—maybe it is true, maybe not. Rather than being a visionary, I think I am particularly good at recognizing brilliant ideas from others. Much more important, I am a planner, and I want to know where I am headed so I can get others on the bus with me, all of us headed to the same place at about the same time. Creating a strategic plan is critical to the stability, growth, and future of any agency. And I firmly believe that with strategic planning the process is as important as the product. You can't lead unless those around you are willing to follow, and there are far too many moving parts in most nonprofit organizations—board, staff, volunteers, donors, clients, and community partners—for you to ever get where you want to be without bringing all of those partners along in your process.

The goal of a strategic plan is to chart an organization's future for the next three, five, eight, or ten years. I have seen strategic-planning processes that have consisted of the executive director's sitting down, writing the plan, and presenting it to the board for ratification, and I have seen processes that have taken years and have employed entire departments. The first method almost never works because there is simply no buy-in from those "on the ground." The second is, in my opinion, too cumbersome; at some point it becomes totally about the process as opposed to the outcomes. I believe most organizational strategic-planning processes should land somewhere in the middle.

The best processes should actively involve all major stakeholders: board, staff, donors, clients, community partners, and volunteers. Up front there should be a statement and a clear understanding of who actually "owns" the process and the final result. In most instances, that should be the board of directors.

When I started at SafePlace they had just completed an extensive strategic plan that had engaged all of the significant constituents in the process. A final focal point of the plan was a need for transitional housing for families leaving shelter. The operational aspects of the plan—how to actually *get* transitional housing—were left up to the staff. Because of that very clear goal, I had buy-in when I suggested that staff become involved in the Travis County Homeless Coalition. It was imperative that I had buy-in because, as I've mentioned, coalition work is very time-consuming. From the strategic plan came the directive for transitional housing, from which came involvement in the Homeless Coalition, from which came the HUD grant and the creation of the SafePlace Supportive Housing Program. Would we have arrived at the same point had we not had the strategic directive, agreed upon by the important stakeholders of the organization? I seriously doubt it.

Be Nimble

Despite all the best planning in the world, sometimes when a window of opportunity opens you have to be ready to jump through it. Merging with the Austin Rape Crisis Center wasn't in any strategic plan when a board member from the Rape Crisis Center met me in a downtown coffee shop and asked if the Center for Battered Women would be open to having a conversation about bringing the two organizations together. It would have been much easier for me, the rest of the staff, and the boards of both agencies if I had simply said no. Instead, I said we should talk about it—and a year later SafePlace, a merger of the Center for Battered Women and the Austin Rape Crisis Center, was born.

Another remarkable demonstration of SafePlace's nimbleness and ability to respond to opportunity and community need resulted in building what would later be named the Kelly White Family Shelter. Homelessness in Austin had become a serious community issue, and Kirk Watson, a visionary and courageous politician and the mayor of Austin at the time, publicly committed to increasing the number of shelter beds. A community task force looked at multiple locations around the city as potential building sites, but all were blocked by strong neighborhood groups and zoning restrictions. The task force, guided by Austin activist and philanthropist Dick Rathgeber, eventually landed on a complex and creative plan that involved moving homeless women and children out of the downtown Salvation Army Shelter in order to free up additional beds for men. The women and children would be relocated to the existing SafePlace shelter, and a new shelter for SafePlace clients would be built on land adjacent to the SafePlace Resource Center and Supportive Housing Program. The brilliance of the plan was undeniable. SafePlace clients and staff, through the Supportive Housing Program, were already active in the local neighborhood association, and the neighbors appreciated both the low profile SafePlace maintained in the neighborhood and the increased police protection our presence brought to the area.

Mayor Watson fought successfully for millions of dollars to build the new facility, but acting on the plan still required the SafePlace board to commit to raising millions more. This came right on the heels of our completing our first capital campaign, and it meant the staff and board would once again be embarking on a time- and resource-intensive building project. Still, it was the absolute best opportunity the agency would ever have to build a model shelter facility—to create a program in a new facility specifically designed to meet residents' needs. The window opened and we leapt.

Remember That It Really Is All about the Money—
Raising It, Spending It, Stewarding It

Whole books are written on fund-raising, but learning a few very important lessons will take you most of the way.

The first and last rule of raising money is "People give to people." People will go to elaborate lengths to avoid having to step up and ask others to give money, but in the end there is no substitute for creating and nurturing personal relationships with donors. People give when someone they trust and believe in asks them personally. They also give when they are asked by someone whom they owe. Figuring out who is the best person to "make the ask" is an important part of raising money. Quid pro quo is alive and well in the world of fund-raising.

Altruism and wanting to do good are also alive and well. I have worked with businesses and corporations too numerous to name that have stepped forward philanthropically because they recognize that by doing so they may assist their employees or their corporate image. Major companies like the Allstate Foundation, Lifetime Television, Kraft Food Brands, Liz Claiborne, and the Body Shop were pioneers in providing funding for domestic-violence programs. Fund-raising is also about figuring out the match, what a donor wants. Listen to and know your donor—what do they care about? Do you remember the old movie *Miracle on 34th Street*, starring Maureen O'Hara and a young Natalie Wood? A kindly gentleman working as a department-store Santa Claus sends customers down the street because Macy's doesn't have the particular item a child wants for Christmas. Santa knew how to listen and try to give people what they needed and wanted.

I said earlier in this book that I am a fixer. I am also a matchmaker. I have set friends up on dates who have now been married for years. I help people find jobs. And I try to listen to what people care about and to find ways in which they can translate that passion into philanthropy. They may not always end up supporting the program I am promoting, but just as it did with the Macy's Santa Claus, the charitable act usually comes back around.

To be effective in making the match, you have to do your research. Know your potential donor, what they care about, their prior giving history to your organization and others, their capacity, and the opportunities available for their support. All too often, fund-raisers leave too much money on the table. They may not have done their research, the wrong person may be making the ask, or they may just be too timid. Early in the first SafePlace capital campaign I flew to Tulsa to visit the Mabee Foundation with one of our campaign steering-committee members, Greg Kozmetsky, a major Austin philanthropist and chairman of the RGK Foundation. Prior to our meeting with the president and chair of the foundation, we sat in the coffee shop on the ground floor of the building. Greg asked, "So, Kelly, how much are we asking for?"

I replied timidly, "Three hundred thousand dollars."

Greg said, "That isn't enough. We're going up there and ask them to give us one million dollars."

I was aghast—not to mention terrified. I had barely learned how to say "one million dollars" without my voice dropping to a whisper. But Greg was confident, and he was right. We were successful in getting a grant of $750,000 from the Mabee Foundation. Had it not been for my friend and mentor Greg, I would have left $450,000 on the table!

I told Greg thank you, and I have been thanking him ever since. You can never say "thank you" too often. Donors and supporters must be stewarded and thanked. Nobody likes a sycophant, but everyone appreciates sincere appreciation.

Keep donors informed about how their funds are being used. Give them opportunities for engagement. Help them to feel good about their investment in your organization. I have invited supportive-housing donors to life skills graduation ceremonies, sent thank-you notes illustrated by children in the child-care program, and provided donors with regular updates and opportunities for involvement.

At SafePlace we regularly asked members of our board and foundation to write thank-you notes to individuals and public officials who provided support for the agency. When Seton Hospital allowed SafePlace to use an entire floor in one of their facilities at no cost for a year while we built the new Resource Center, we sent thank-you notes to the hospital CEO. He later told me that he had never been so profusely thanked by so many people, and that everyone at Seton felt immensely appreciated for their contribution to SafePlace.

Major donors will want to connect with the leadership of the agency — both volunteer and paid. Donors are making an investment in your organization, and savvy investors care about whom and what they are investing in. But all of the personal requests, listening, research, and stewardship won't count for much if the organization doesn't have a viable, credible product: a mission that matters and services that are effective and accountable to the community.

Be a Leader

Leadership matters. I was a good manager long before I was a good leader. And let me be quick to add that being a good leader is a goal that always beckons and is never quite attained. But I had the additional obstacle of needing to gain the understanding that leadership is important. In my mind, leadership was commensurate with power, and power was something people abused.

When most battered-women's programs began they were based on an egalitarian, nonhierarchical model of shared leadership. All decisions were made by consensus, all staff drew the same salary, and, even while promoting so-called empowerment, they actively pulled back from promoting women as individually powerful. This was very much the organizational culture that was in place when I first started working in the movement. And as a formerly battered woman I think I was particularly sensitive to any hint of abuse of power on my part.

Two years into my job as executive director of Safehouse, in Denver, and almost seven years into my career as an executive director, I met with three of my board members for lunch at an upscale restaurant near my office. I remember immediately recognizing that they had clearly orchestrated beforehand how they were going to talk with me. The topic was leadership. They told me they thought I was a good manager, that I attended well to the administration of the organization, but they wanted me to step up as a leader.

I was confused by their request. I tried to explain that leaders weren't acceptable in the battered-women's movement — to be a leader was a bad thing. They insisted differently, that to be a leader was not inherently sinister. Following our conversation I spent time thinking and studying and observing. I have been fascinated with the subject of leadership ever since. I saw that there were indeed many leaders in the battered-women's movement. Perhaps they weren't designated as such by title or position, but they were leaders nevertheless. I tried to figure out what kind of leadership seemed to be positive and effective and the type of leader I would like to be.

I found that I had no interest in being a charismatic leader: someone who needs and expects to be out front and followed blindly because of the force of her personality. Some charismatic leaders are tremendously effective, but the success of their organization is tied to one individual. I am not suited to being a charismatic leader, nor is it my goal to create and build an organization that is dependent on my continued participation. I want to be able to step away knowing that I have helped to create something that is sustainable beyond my tenure.

Many leaders have been designated so by their titles and positions, not necessarily by their leadership qualities. Examples are abundant in businesses, families, government, and academia. This type of leadership measures an individual's power and decision-making authority by their rank or title rather than by their ability to motivate and encourage the character, courage, creativity, and skills of the individuals in the organization. Again, I don't think this is an effective long-term form of leadership. At its worst it can be damaging.

Battered-women's programs, so aware of the dynamics of power and control, are not immune to abuse of power. I have seen so-called leaders require staff to lie to cover their actions as they abuse their power by engaging in sexual relationships with clients. Such a relationship, because of the imbalance of power between the involved parties, can never be considered anything other than coerced. I have seen designated leaders threaten staff with the fear of losing a job, or worse, as they compel them to lie about finances, programming, and other staff.

Leaders whom I admire and try to emulate have several things in common: They show up, commit to the journey, have the courage to make unpopular decisions, and honor the integrity of the decision-making process. I have worked hard at being the type of leader who thinks beyond the horizon. An elderly gentleman whom I knew many years ago in Fort Worth, Texas, told me he had lost his second-term race for mayor because he was a better statesman than politician. The difference between the two, he explained, was that "a politician works for the next election, while a statesman is working for the next generation." He certainly understood about thinking beyond the horizon.

Leadership qualities such as personal responsibility, truth, respect for the individual, and courage have applications throughout our work and social lives. Mahatma Gandhi, one of the greatest leaders of the twentieth century, wielded tremendous power based solely on the willingness of people to follow his lead. The Indian people were willing to serve him because his life was devoted to serving them.

The leaders I admire and work to emulate never accept the status quo. The statement "That's the way we have always done it" is absolute anathema to me. If it's not the right way, the smart way, the ethical way, then let's figure out how to fix it — fix the laws, fix the people, fix the process. It may take a lifetime, but there isn't much that can't be changed.

I have also learned to choose my battles. When we were building the new SafePlace Resource Center I was appalled to learn that the city building code dictated the specific number of men's restrooms and urinals regardless of the usage of the building. I protested long and hard, based on the fact that the building was primarily to be used by women and children, and that men are perfectly capable of using a toilet whereas women are highly inconvenienced by having to use a urinal. The architects finally made me see that if I chose to continue this battle with the city, which I would probably eventually win, I would delay our construction by years. I needed to let this battle go. I did. But just by my mentioning it in this book you know that it still sticks in my craw.

My goal is to provide consistent and transparent leadership. I try to communicate constructively and directly. I'm not always successful, but it is my goal. I also try to admit when I am wrong, which happens far too often. Unfortunately, when I am right I also have the tendency to say, "I told you so."

I wasn't a cheerleader in high school, but I have sure found that I sometimes need to be a cheerleader in my work. My role has often been as the person who is out front telling others we can raise the money, finish the building, convince the board, change the policy, or take just one more client. I am often the one saying, "Yes, we can do this," even when I am up at night wondering how in the world we can possibly do it.

Donna Shalala, then U.S. Secretary of Health and Human Services, spoke at the groundbreaking when SafePlace completed renovation of its single women's shelter. Her advance person came the day before to make certain everything was ready, and he was horrified to discover that the site was still under construction, with building debris and construction equipment littering the grounds. It was clear to everyone that he feared for his job. When he showed up the next morning with Secretary Shalala he was amazed to find the building clean, painted, and decorated, and all of the construction debris and equipment gone. What he didn't know was that things were hidden behind the back privacy fence, the nicely made beds had no mattresses, and every closet and drawer was packed with paint cans and stray nails. I knew when to say, "We don't need to make this perfect, we just need to get it done." And we did.

I was in there helping to clean the parking lot and toss things over the back fence. I will never ask someone to do something I am not willing to do myself. I will and have cleaned toilets, told people they are fired, talked with difficult clients, written grants, and answered the phones. When a VISTA volunteer announced to me that her contract said she didn't have to make copies, I said, "Fine, give it to me. I make copies."

One of my absolute favorite stories has to do with Laura Bush, then first lady of Texas. Mrs. Bush, always a lovely and gracious woman, served on the Board of Trustees of the SafePlace Foundation. We were hosting an open house prior to moving clients into our new supportive-housing apartments, and we were, as always, rushing at the last possible moment to get everything clean and finished for the occasion. Just moments prior to the beginning of the event, dressed in my best business suit and heels, I was scrubbing the toilets — it had to be done — when the first lady's security detail arrived at the door, followed quickly by Laura herself, just as I peeled off my rubber gloves and stowed the toilet brush under the cabinet.

I don't always need or want to be the leader. Depending on the situation, someone else may provide more effective leadership. Leadership is like a relay; the baton regularly gets handed off to a person who is fresh or better prepared for a particular leg of the race. Creating new and more diverse leadership for the next generation is core to the work of ending violence against women. Ultimately, domestic-violence programs are not about providing shelter or supportive housing, answering the crisis line, or providing legal advocacy. Ultimately, this work is about broadening and deepening the leadership in the movement so that everyone has an expectation of respect for themselves and one another. Advancing the leadership of women and girls is key to a rebalanced globe.

14

our work
isn't done

The twentieth century will be remembered as a century marked by violence. Less visible, but even more widespread, is the legacy of day-to-day, individual suffering. It is the pain of children who are abused by people who should protect them, women injured or humiliated by violent partners, elderly persons maltreated by their caregivers.... No country, no city, no community is immune. But neither are we powerless against it.... Violence can be prevented. Violent cultures can be turned around.... In order to ensure this, we must be tireless in our efforts not only to attain peace, justice, and prosperity for country, but for communities and members of the same family. We must address the roots of violence. Only then will we transform the past century's legacy from a crushing burden into a cautionary lesson.

— Nelson Mandela

WHEN I FELT EMPOWERED TO STEP FORTH AND TALK ABOUT the abuse in my first marriage without self-blame or fear of being labeled weak or culpable, I created a new norm in my world and in the understanding of those around me. I once sat in my office with two potential donors, including Dick Rathgeber, an Austin philanthropist who helped to raise millions of dollars for SafePlace. Dick said to me in his deep West Texas twang, "But what about these guys? They are going to continue to prey on weak women until we do something about them."

My response surprised him. "Weak? I don't think so!"

The other donor, a woman, said, "Do we look weak to you?"

Dick was incredulous when both of us told him that we had been battered women. I am willing to bet that he has never again referred to battered women as "weak."

Still, Dick was exactly right in one respect: We will never end violence against women by focusing on women alone. We must engage men and boys; we must work to change the community systems, rigid gender stereotypes, and cultures of oppression that foster abuse. We must drain the swamp in which all of the attitudes are bred that promote gender violence.

In the nonprofit world a tension always exists between investing in direct services like additional shelter beds or counseling, and allocating scarce resources to programs addressing the prevention of bullying, sexual harassment, or teen-dating violence. The further step of advocating for policy change is usually distasteful to funders. I don't think it is possible to choose between intervention, prevention, and social change. We shouldn't be forced into making such choices — sufficient resources should be available to address all the issues. When the barn is burning down you obviously have to put out the fire, but that doesn't mean you abandon fire-prevention efforts such as educating people and improving building codes. The same should be true of domestic violence. And as with fire prevention, the savings in lives and dollars that are realized through efforts to prevent domestic violence are incalculable. Imagine the reduction in costs in areas such as law enforcement, the courts, prisons, health care, and almost all of the seemingly intractable human-service problems if we could reduce domestic violence in the United States by even 10 percent.

Where and how do we begin to drain the swamp? At SafePlace we started with prevention programs in local high schools, but we quickly realized that even high school was too late for primary prevention. Domestic violence was already a fact of life for too many of the students we talked with.

Teen–Dating Violence–Prevention Programs

In the mid-1990s, Barri Rosenbluth, director of Expect Respect, the SafePlace teen-dating violence-prevention program, wanted to apply for a grant through the Centers for Disease Control and Prevention (CDC) to address violence prevention at the elementary-school level. As the mother of a grade-school-age daughter and two middle-school sons, I admit I was reticent. I simply couldn't see how we could, or why we would need to, address gender violence at such a young age. My opinion changed one morning while I was braiding my daughter's hair. She talked innocently about what was happening to her on the playground each day. Megan said that at recess she sat with the playground monitor rather than going out to play with the other children. When I asked why, her response astonished me.

"Mom, Mitch chases me all over the playground trying to kiss me, and I don't like it, so I just sit and talk with Ms. Donnell."

"Have you tried telling Ms. Donnell that you don't like it when Mitch chases you?"

"Yes, but Ms. Donnell says he just does that because he likes me, so it's okay."

My second-grade daughter was being taught that when a boy chased her with unwanted advances it was her responsibility to change her behavior, and that when she went to an authority to ask for assistance none was forthcoming. I seriously doubt that Mitch was a nascent sexual predator, and I remember engaging in the same kinds of playground games when I was a child. But I suddenly understood why and how SafePlace could engage in domestic violence–prevention programs with elementary-school students. This was an opportunity to change behaviors and attitudes before they escalated to teen-dating violence.

SafePlace, together with the University of Texas School of Social Work, developed a research-based program designed to evaluate reduction in bullying behavior in fifth-grade students. We utilized the Bully Proofing curriculum developed by Nan Stein, senior researcher at Wellesley College. Our goal was to emphasize bullying as one element on a continuum that includes sexual harassment, sexual assault, stalking, and dating/domestic violence.

Most of us know the toll that bullying takes on children. It has been shrugged off as "kids being kids," but it is a serious problem. As many as 7 percent of eighth-grade students in the United States stay home at least once a month because of their fear of bullies. And the effects of bullying are grim for the offender. One study shows that 60 percent of children identified as bullies in sixth through ninth grades had at least one criminal conviction by age twenty-four.[1] Studies have found that many of the recent school shooters experienced severe and long-term bullying. When someone feels incredibly helpless or powerless, they can take extreme action to try to regain their power.

Unfortunately, violence-prevention programs haven't typically addressed the problem of bullying. Generally, they have consisted of conflict-resolution and anger-management strategies, neither of which prevent bullying or address the underlying issue of power imbalances that eventually translate into more generalized violence. Additionally, most research shows that bullying starts in early elementary school and peaks in late elementary and middle school. By high school the behaviors have often progressed to include dating violence or harassment of gay and lesbian teens and others considered vulnerable or powerless.

Recognizing that something is wrong and then taking proactive steps toward change is difficult, particularly in large organizations like public school systems. We were eventually able to show significant decreases in bullying behaviors by implementing a whole-school approach. All school personnel were engaged, from teachers, administrators, and parents to playground monitors and bus drivers. Had my daughter's school received the training, Ms. Donnell would have learned to intervene between Mitch and Megan.

The first step for both adults and children is to recognize bullying when it occurs; the next step is to intervene. An important part of the Bully Proofing curriculum is training and encouraging students to be "courageous bystanders." Intervening in bullying becomes everyone's responsibility; bullying isn't simply regarded as a problem between victim and offender. Students are taught to step in with peer support and say, "Your behavior isn't okay. Stop it." It is enormously powerful for students to step forward and say this as a group.

We have been told since we were young that "no one likes a tattletale." What is the difference between tattling and reporting bullying? The primary difference lies in the purpose. When a child tattles, she does so in order to get the other child into trouble. When a child reports an incident or difficult situation to a teacher or parent and asks for help, they should be listened to. My daughter, Megan, should have been listened to when she asked the playground monitor for assistance with the little boy who bothered her. She wasn't tattling; she was asking for a responsible adult to intervene to make the playground feel like a safe place for her. Too often, when students go to adults for help with bullying incidents, the students feel they aren't taken seriously. They are admonished to work it out on their own, or they are told, "That's just normal," or, as in Megan's case, "Boys will be boys."

When we first started training people in the Bully Proofing curriculum, we quickly realized that adult perceptions of gender roles could interfere with teaching children about behaviors that should raise red flags. In an early group training, when given a hypothetical situation in which a boy wouldn't leave a girl alone, calling her incessantly, following her, and tracking her every move, one teacher was overheard remarking to another, "I wish some man would care about me that much." Having been the recipient of that kind of stalking and obsessive control, I clearly understand that it isn't love; it is an attempt at ownership.

I recently read *Twilight*, the phenomenally successful young-adult novel by Stephenie Meyer. In it, the shy, awkward Bella falls in love with Edward, a handsome, sensitive vampire who lives in the cloud-covered mountains with his adopted family of fellow vampires. I, too, was entranced by the romance and the forbidden love, but I was also very troubled by the obsessive behavior that is portrayed in the book as "true love." Edward snuck into Bella's room at night and, unknown to her, watched her as she slept. This was eerily similar to my former husband Jay's behavior; he would watch me through my window as I slept. At the end of the book Edward saves Bella's life from an evil vampire and shows his love by tasting her blood but resisting the urge to take all of it—or, metaphorically, resisting his desire to go all the way—while Bella lies unconscious in his arms. It is a modern-day fairy tale that perpetuates all of the so-called romantic myths that have been so destructive to the development of healthy relationships between men and women for many generations.

How can we change perceptions of gender roles unless we create new, healthy role models and stereotypes? How can we show young people that love is not expressed through obsessive control? We need to portray girls as powerful and in control of their destinies and boys as gentle and respectful of girls and women. We need to create new expectations in both sexes of what it means to be powerful and male or powerful and female.

Numerous teen-dating violence programs have been developed that strive to promote safe and healthy relationships. Expect Respect, the nationally recognized program created by SafePlace, has been replicated across the country, but still only a tiny percentage of teens are introduced to these ideas, particularly when compared to the massive reach of today's media. Teens must first learn to identify love and abuse. Young men must also learn to recognize, name, and deal with their feelings nondestructively. Usually, anger is the tip of an iceberg, masking feelings of hurt, humiliation, frustration, and fear. Boys have learned at home, through the popular culture, and in institutionalized settings such as schools that it is acceptable to vent their anger against women and girls.

Men as Allies

Ending violence against women will only be accomplished with women and men working together. Men *are not* the enemy. My sons, father, husband, and brothers all have actively worked to be a part of the solution. Men are every bit as trapped by the stereotype of the all-powerful, controlling male as women are trapped by the image of the weak, submissive female.

Years ago I was involved in efforts to create an all-male, honorary advisory group associated with SafePlace called ManPower. The group was a huge success; men vied for the honor of publicly standing for respectful, healthy relationships. We were able to attract high-profile, influential, and affluent men to affiliate their names with our organization. The editor of the editorial page of the daily newspaper, the *Austin-American Statesman*, said, "How in the world could I say no?"

Early in the process we discovered we needed to be careful whom we asked to participate. We had finalized our list of invitees. It was a good, diverse list, broadly representative of various parts of the community, including corporate and nonprofit entities, governmental agencies, academia, health care, philanthropic organizations, and varied religious and racial groups. The next day we would start making the calls. That evening, I opened the latest *Time* magazine. My eyes were immediately drawn to a headline, "Men Behaving Badly." Beneath it was a photo of Neil Bush, an Austin resident at the time and the brother of then Texas governor George W. Bush. Neil happened to be on our list of invitees. The article detailed a string of questionable personal and business decisions he had made. I am not saying he would never be suitable for inclusion on a list of men supportive of ending domestic violence, but given the article's appearance that particular week in a national publication, timing was certainly not on his side. We removed him from the list of prospective invitees.

We also created a purely fund-raising vehicle called Men Who Love Women. For a hefty price, a man could be publicly recognized as standing in support of ending violence against women. Some people have said that the name sounds "sexist" or "homophobic." My response was to point out that the gay men I know like women better than almost anyone else. The word "love" doesn't have to connote sex. And we *must* publicly engage men's voices as a part of the solution.

Men who hold women down also hold themselves and their families down. Men who support and elevate women also elevate themselves, their families, and their communities.

Elevating Women and Girls

To end violence against women and girls we must elevate all women. Private and public sectors must partner to create opportunities for economic security, access to health care, and affordable child care. The basic trends that have impacted women historically are still very much in play. "Women's jobs" pay less, and women continue to shoulder the majority of family-care responsibilities, a big piece of which is child care. Single working mothers continue to report that a majority of their income goes toward paying for child care while they work, and that a major cause of missing work is a breakdown in those child-care plans.

Currently, seven out of ten mothers in the United States with children under age eighteen work outside of the home. Yet, even adjusted for time away from the workplace to have children, women still earn only seventy-eight cents for every dollar that men earn, which in 2007 averaged out to an annual gap of $10,000. Women of color come up even shorter.[3] The National Committee on Pay Equity reports that over a lifetime a woman with only a high school diploma earns $700,000 less than a man with the same level of education. The gap is even greater between women and men who hold college or professional degrees: $1.2 million and $2 million respectively.[4]

As a nation we have been appalled by the treatment of women in Afghanistan and many other countries around the globe; yet injustices still exist in the United States. My work and life experience have shown me that we can only end violence against women and girls by simultaneously working to create opportunities and equity for women.

It is important to tell women's stories, to identify and advocate for public policy that will provide increased opportunities and will promote women's work as valuable and worthy of greater pay. Advancing the cause of women involves engaging women and men of all races and classes to identify and create strategies for change in their local communities.

We can begin by fostering a mindset in which women are no longer viewed as long-suffering victims or noble survivors, but rather as leaders empowered to take initiative and solve problems. It is time to change the dialogue. Leymah Gbowee founded Women of Liberia Mass Action for Peace, which demanded a nonviolent resolution to the bloody civil war that had torn Liberia apart for years. In a country where it was estimated that two out of every three women had been raped, the activists risked assault and even slaughter to protest the regime of President Charles Taylor. They were a key force in the peaceful exile of Taylor and the election of Ellen Johnson Sirleaf, the first elected female president of an African country. Their extraordinary story was told in the award-winning documentary *Pray the Devil Back to Hell,* produced by Abigail Disney.

Ending Violence One Person at a Time

We must always remember that it was one courageous woman, Leymah Gbowee, who started what became a movement in Liberia. We end violence one person at a time. Each individual, man or woman, who turns away from violence brings others along.

Joan Carter, longtime SafePlace legal advocate and herself a survivor of horrific abuse at the hands of her ex-husband, a wealthy Texas businessman, recently spoke of a survivor who has stepped up to help others.

One morning we had a protective-order hearing between Susan and Bill. Susan is a current SafePlace client who had been befriended by Alice, a former SafePlace client. Alice had been a regular attendee in the support group I facilitated back in 1996.

Alice and her daughter had lived in their car at one point before getting into the shelter. I had loved watching Alice find herself, make new friends in the support group, and regain her self-esteem. She worked at multiple jobs to get back on her feet and into school.

Most important, she was living a safe, abuse-free life. Her teenage daughter saw her mom grow into a really strong role model.

Bill threatened to kill both Susan and Alice, but Susan was able to "borrow" strength and support from Alice. During one assault, Susan ran out of a hotel room and called on Alice to come rescue her.

Both women were very strong on the stand. Alice in particular was as perfect a witness as a prosecutor could want. She was concise, to the point, and nonargumentative — cool and in control. Later she admitted that she was shaking as she testified while Bill sat in the courtroom and stared at her with open hostility.

It was a long, contested hearing, but with Alice coming forward of her own volition as a witness, the dilemma of "he said versus she said" was eliminated for the judge. The protective order was granted.

This is clearly a case of a formerly battered woman taking to heart the concept of "carrying the torch" by helping another woman who was struggling and in danger. Both of these women had received death threats, yet they still came forward. It gave me chills as I thought of the courage it takes to face an abuser in court, especially when he is not in jail and continues to pose a threat.

I was so proud of Alice — I felt like a new mom who had just given birth. I had witnessed a miraculous transformation of two women who had found strength with the support and caring of each other and of SafePlace. Besides Alice's breaking the chain of abuse in her life and her daughter's life, who knows how many women she has helped since 1996. She is my hero.

Joan herself is a hero to many. I once presented a SafePlace credit card at an Office Depot, and the store employee, noting the organization's name on the card, said to me, "Joan Carter saved my life. She is my hero." I have heard numerous people in the community say that about her.

I wish I could tell the stories of all the heroes I have met. What I have learned from them is that although we can't turn away from the hard work of changing policy and cultural norms, we also must count our successes one woman, one child, and one family at a time. We will not end the need for battered-women's shelters, twenty-four-hour crisis lines, or protective orders in my lifetime. Our vision is to end violence against women and to put ourselves out of business, but it simply won't happen in this generation. The issues are too complex and the problems too intractable. Still, we must recognize and celebrate the individual lives saved, the children who learn how to live with peace, and the heroes who do the work.

When I stood under the tent as the new shelter was being dedicated and was told that it had been named in my honor, I was humbled to hear people say I was a hero. What I do know is that I have helped to transform the dialogue. I have been blessed to help women redefine themselves from victims to survivors, leaders, and agents of change.

❧ *Notes* ❧

Chapter 2: Surviving and Speaking Out: Building My Life Free from Violence

1. K. J. Wilson, *When Violence Begins at Home,* 1st ed. (Alameda, CA: Hunter House Publishers, 1997), 251–52.

Chapter 3: Defining the Problem of Domestic Abuse

1. Megan Twohey and Liam Ford, "The Law Didn't Save Her," *Chicago Tribune,* 16 March 2008, http://www.chicagotribune.com.
2. Federal Bureau of Investigation, "Crime in the United States: 2000—Uniform Crime Reports," 2001, http://www.fbi.gov/about-us/cjis/ucr/crime-in-the-u.s/2000.
3. National Coalition Against Domestic Violence, "Homicide and Domestic Violence Facts: When Men Murder Women," 2004, http://www.ncadv.org/files/WhenMenMurderWomen2004_.pdf.
4. Vivian C. Fox, "Historical Perspective on Violence Against Women," *Journal of International Women's Studies* 4, no. 1 (2002): 15.
5. K. J. Wilson, *When Violence Begins at Home,* 1st ed. (Alameda, CA: Hunter House Publishers, 1997), 250.
6. Will Durant, *The Greatest Minds and Ideas of All Time*, comp. John Little (New York: Simon and Schuster, 2002), 8–30.
7. Aristotle, *Politics*, Book 1, Chapter V (Seattle, WA: CreateSpace, 2010).
8. http://www.quotes.net/authors/Plato.
9. R. E. Dobash and R. P. Dobash, *Violence Against Wives, A Case Against Patriarchy* (New York: Free Press, 1979), 37.
10. Wilson, *When Violence Begins at Home*, 264.
11. D. Rogers (London, 1642) in Anthony Fletcher, *Gender, Sex and Subordination in England, 1500–1800* (New Haven, CT: Yale University Press, 1995), 74.
12. Ibid., 192.
13. Linda K. Kerber, Jane S. De Hart, and Cornelia H. Dayton, *Women's America: Refocusing the Past*, 4th ed. (New York: Oxford University Press, 1995), 13.
14. Susan Brownmiller, *Against Our Will: Men, Women and Rape* (New York: Ballantine, 1975), 16–19.
15. Andrea Dworkin, *Woman Hating* (New York: Plume, 1974), 101–103.

16. D. K. Stein, "Women to Burn: Suttee as a Normative Institution," in *Femicide: The Politics of Woman Killing,* ed. H. Radford and D. E. H. Russell (New York: Twayne Publishers, 1992), 62.

17. Wilson, *When Violence Begins at Home,* 272.

18. L. Narashimhan, *Sati: Widow Burning in India* (New York: Anchor Books, 1990), 61–73.

19. Afif Sartar, "Hitmen Charge $100 a Victim as Basra Honour Killings Rise," *The Observer,* 30 November 2008, http://www.guardian.co.uk/world /2008/nov/30/iraq-honor-killings-women.

20. Joan Chittister, *When Violence Against Women Is Honorable, Religious, and Legal,* National Catholic Reporter Conversation Cafe (ncrcafe.org), 24 May 2007.

21. Sherry Karabin, "Infanticide, Abortions Responsible for 60 Million Girls Missing in Asia," 13 June 2007, FoxNews.com, http://www.foxnews.com /story/0,2933,281722,00.html.

22. Sonja Wolte, "Ending Violence Against Women and Girls—Protecting Human Rights," Deutsche Gesellschaft fur Technische Zusammenarbeit (GTZ), Eschborn, December 2003, http://www2.gtz.de/dokumente/bib /05-1048.pdf.

23. Wolte, "Ending Violence Against Women and Girls."

24. "Family Violence Statistics: Including Statistics on Strangers and Acquaintances." US Department of Justice, Bureau of Justice Statistics, 2005, http://www.ojp.usdoj.gov/bjs/pub/pdf/fvs.pdf.

25. "Adverse Health Conditions and Health Risk Behaviors Associated with Intimate Partner Violence, Morbidity and Mortality," Weekly Report, 8 February 2008, Centers for Disease Control and Prevention, http://www .cdc.gov/mmwr/preview/mmwrhtml/mm5705a1.htm.

26. "Family Violence Statistics: Including Statistics on Strangers and Acquaintances," US Department of Justice, Bureau of Justice Statistics, 2005, http://www.ojp.usdoj.gov/bjs/pub/pdf/fvs.pdf.

27. *Examining the Work of State Courts, 1995: A National Perspective from the Court Statistics Project,* National Center for the State Courts, 1996.

28. Patricia Tjaden and Nancy Thoennes, *Full Report of the Prevalence, Incidence, and Consequences of Violence Against Women: Findings from the National Violence Against Women Survey* (Washington, DC: National Institute of Justice, 2000), http://www.ncjrs.gov/pdffiles1/nij/183781.pdf.

29. L. K. Hamberger and C. G. Use, "Men's and Women's Use of Intimate Partner Violence in Clinical Samples," *Violence Against Women* 8, no. 11 (2002): 1301–31.

30. Tjaden and Thoennes, *Full Report of the Prevalence, Incidence, and Consequences.*

31. The National Domestic Violence Hotline, http://www.thehotline.org/is -this-abuse/am-I-being-abused-2.

32. US Advisory Board on Child Abuse and Neglect, *A Nation's Shame: Fatal Child Abuse and Neglect in the United States,* Fifth Report, US Advisory Board on Child Abuse and Neglect, US Department of Health and Human Services, 1995, http://ican-ncfr.org/documents/Nations-Shame.pdf

33. Murray A. Strauss, Richard J.Gelles, and Christine Smith, *Physical Violence in American Families: Risk Factors and Adaptations to Violence in 8,145 Families* (New Brunswick, NJ: Transaction Publishers, 1990), 113–32.

34. Janet Carter and Susan Schechter, *Child Abuse and Domestic Violence: Creating Community Partnerships for Safe Families,* Family Violence Prevention Fund, 1997, http://www.mincava.umn.edu/link/documents/fvpfl /fvpfl.shtml.

35. P. A. Fazzone, J. K. Holton, and B. G. Reed, "Substance Abuse Treatment and Domestic Violence: Treatment Improvement Protocol," US Department of Health and Human Services Publication No (SMA) 9703163, Rockville, MD, http://www.ncbi.nlm.nih.gov/bookshelf/br.fcgi?book =hssamhsatip&part=A46882.

36. *Making the Link: Domestic Violence and Alcohol and Other Drugs,* US Department of Health and Human Services and SAMHSA's National Clearinghouse for Alcohol and Drug Information, http://roar.nevadaprc.org /resource/docs/0000/0657/DomesticViolence.pdf.

37. James J. Collins and Donna L. Spencer, *Linkage of Domestic Violence and Substance Abuse Services: Research in Brief,* US Department of Justice, 2002. http://www.ncjrs.gov/pdffiles1/nij/grants/194122.pdf.

38. V. J. Felitti, et al., "Relationship of Childhood Abuse and Household Dysfunction to Many of the Leading Causes of Death in Adults. The Adverse Childhood Experiences (ACE) Study," *American Journal of Preventive Medicine* 14, no. 4 (1998): 245–58.

39. Fazzone, Holton, and Reed, *Substance Abuse Treatment and Domestic Violence.*

40. Collins and Spencer, *Linkage of Domestic Violence and Substance Abuse Services.*

41. Patricia Tjaden and Nancy Thoennes, "Prevalence, Incidence, and Consequences of Violence Against Women: Findings from the National Violence Against Women Survey," National Institute of Justice, Research in Brief, November 1998, http://www.ncjrs.gov/pdffiles/172837.pdf.

42. Shannan M. Catalano, "Crime Victimization, 2004," National Crime Victimization Survey (Washington DC: US Department of Justice, Bureau of Justice Statistics, 2005), http://www.rainn.org/get-information/statistics /sexual-assault-victims.

43. H. N. Snyder, *Sexual Assault of Young Children As Reported to Law Enforcement: Victim, Incident, and Offender Characteristics* (NCJ 182990) (Washington, DC: US Department of Justice, 2000), http://www.eric.ed.gov /PDFS/ED446834.pdf.

44. Etienne G. Krug, et al., eds., *World Report on Violence and Health*, Chapter Six, "Sexual Violence," (Geneva, Switzerland: World Health Organization, 2002), http://whqlibdoc.who.int/publications/2002/9241545615_chap6 _eng.pdf.

45. American Medical Association, "Sexual Assault in America: Guidelines on Sexual Assault," (Chicago, IL: AMA, 1995).

Chapter 4: Generations

1. Break the Cycle, "Startling Statistics," 2006, http://www.breakthecycle.org /HTML%20files/1_4a_startstatis.htm.

2. C. L. Whitfield, et al., "Violent Childhood Experiences and the Risk of Intimate Partner Violence in Adults: Assessment in a Large Health Maintenance Organization," *Journal of Interpersonal Violence* 18, no. 2 (2003): 166–85.

3. K. A. McDonnell, A.C. Gielen, and P. O'Campo, "Does HIV Status Make a Difference in the Experience of Lifetime Abuse? Descriptions of Lifetime Abuse and Its Context among Low-income Urban Women," *Journal of Urban Health* 80, no. 3 (2003), 494–500.

Chapter 5: Who Is at Risk?

1. Denise Hines and Kathleen Malley-Morrison, *Family Violence in the United States* (Thousand Oaks, CA: Sage Publications, 2005), 280.

2. Ibid., 282.

3. Dan Sorenson, "Hate Crimes Against People with Disabilities," 2001, http://www.cavnet2.org/partnersdetails.cfm?DocID=2489&partnerid =1228.

4. I. S. Horon and D. Cheng, "Enhanced Surveillance for Pregnancy-Associated Mortality—Maryland, 1993–1998," *The Journal of the American Medical Association* 285, no. 11 (21 March 2001): 1455–59.

5. Carole Warshaw and Holly Barnes, "Domestic Violence, Mental Health and Trauma, Research Highlights," April, 2003, http://www.dvmhpi.org /research/publications.htm.

6. K. T. Mueser, et al., "Trauma and Posttraumatic Stress Disorder in Severe Mental Illness," *Journal of Consulting and Clinical Psychology* 66 (1998): 493–99.

7. S. N. Goodwin, S. Changler, and J. Meisel, *Violence Against Women: The Role of Welfare Reform, Final Report*, National Criminal Justice Reference

System, 11 April 2003, http://www.ncjrs.gov/pdffiles1/nij/grants/205792 .pdf.

8. M. Schwartz, W. Abramson, and H. Kamper, "A National Survey on the Accessibility of Domestic Violence and Sexual Assault Services to Women with Disabilities," unpublished raw data, 2003, Austin, TX: SafePlace.

9. Patricia Tjaden and Nancy Thoennes, *Extent, Nature, and Consequences of Intimate Partner Violence: Findings from the National Violence Against Women Survey*, US Department of Justice, Office of Justice Programs, 2000, 4–5, http://www.ncjrs.gov/pdffiles1/nij/181867.pdf.

10. K. J. Wilson, *When Violence Begins at Home*, 1st ed. (Alameda, CA: Hunter House Publishers, 1997), 119.

11. Hines and Malley-Morrison, *Family Violence in the United States*, 53.

12. R. L. Burgess, J. M. Leone, and S. M. Kleinbaum, "Social and Ecological Issues in Violence Toward Children," in *Case Studies in Family Violence*, 2nd ed., eds. R. T. Ammerman and M. Hersen (New York: Plenum, 2000), 15–38.

13. M. R. Rank, "The Effect of Poverty on America's Families: Assessing Our Research Knowledge," *Journal of Family Issues* 22 (2001): 885.

14. M. L. Benson and G. L. Fox, *When Violence Hits Home: How Economics and Neighborhood Play a Role*, Research in Brief (Washington: National Institute of Justice, US Department of Justice, 2004), ii, http://www.ncjrs .gov/pdffiles1/nij/205004.pdf.

15. R. K. Lee, V. L. Sanders Thompson, and M. B. Mechanic, "Intimate Partner Violence and Women of Color: A Call for Innovations," *American Journal of Public Health* 92 (April 2002): 530–34.

16. Tjaden and Thoennes, *Extent, Nature, and Consequences of Intimate Partner Violence.*

17. Mary Dutton, Leslye Orloff, and Giselle Aguilar Hass, "Characteristics of Help-Seeking Behaviors, Resources, and Services Needs of Battered Immigrant Latinas: Legal and Policy Implications," *Georgetown Journal on Poverty Law and Policy* 7, no. 245 (2000): 245–305, http://endabuse.org /userfiles/file/children_and_families/Immigrant.pdf.

18. Patricia Tjaden and Nancy Thoennes, *Full Report of the Prevalence, Incidence and Consequences of Violence Against Women: Findings from the National Violence Against Women Survey* (Washington, D.C.: National Institute of Justice and the Centers for Disease Control and Prevention, 2000), http://www.ncjrs.org/pdffiles1/nij/183781.pdf.

19. R. J. Gelles, G. D. Wolfner, and R. Lackner, "Men Who Batter: The Risk Markers," *Violence Update* 4 (1994): 1–10.

20. T. E. Moffitt and A. Caspi, *Findings about Partner Violence from the Dunedin Multidisciplinary Health and Development Study: Research in Brief*

(Washington, D.C.: National Institute of Justice, US Department of Justice, 1999), 2.

21. Richard J. Gelles, *Intimate Violence in Families* (Thousand Oaks, CA: Sage Publications, 1997), 85.

Chapter 6: Survivors: Much More than Former Victims

1. Patricia Tjaden and Nancy Thoennes, *Extent, Nature, and Consequences of Rape Victimization: Findings from the National Violence Against Women Survey, Special Report* (Washington, DC: National Institute of Justice and the Centers for Disease Control and Prevention, 2006), http://www.ncjrs .gov/pdffiles1/nij/210346.pdf.

2. T. Styron and R. Janoff-Bulman, "Childhood Attachment and Abuse: Long-term Effects on Adults," *Journal of Child Abuse and Neglect* 21, no. 10 (October 1997): 1015–23.

3. B. Benard, *Fostering Resiliency in Kids: Protective Factors in the Family, School, and Community,* ED 335 781 (San Francisco, CA: Far West Laboratory for Educational Research and Development, 1991), 6.

Chapter 7: The Batterer

1. US Department of Justice, *National Crime Victim Survey,* 1995.

2. University of Cincinnati's School of Social Work Findings, presented at the Tenth International Conference on Family Violence, San Diego, CA, September 2005.

3. Minnesota Center Against Violence and Abuse (MINCAVA), "Guidelines for Men Who Batter Programs," 1997, http://www.mincava.umn.edu /documents/pwwmwb2/pwwmwb2.html.

4. Jane E. Brody, "Battered Women Face Pit Bulls and Cobras," *New York Times,* 17 March 1998, Health section.

5. Megan Twohey, "Too Many to Stop," *Chicago Tribune,* 12 March 2009, 1.

6. D.G. Saunders and R.M. Hamill, "Violence Against Women: Synthesis of Research on Offender Interventions," National Institute of Justice, June 2003, http://www.ncjrs.gov/pdffiles1/nij/grants/201222.pdf.

Chapter 8: The Youngest Survivors: Children and Domestic Violence

1. SafePlace in-house document, 2008.

2. SafePlace in-house document, 2008.

3. SafePlace in-house document, 2008.

4. B.E. Carlson, "Children's Observations of Interparental Violence," in *Battered Women and Their Families,* ed. A.R. Roberts (New York: Springer, 1984), 147–67.

5. Joy D. Osofsky, "The Impact of Violence on Children: The Future of Children," *Domestic Violence and Children* 9, no. 3 (winter 1999): 38.

6. C. Roustit, et al., "Exposure to Interparental Violence and Psychosocial Maladjustment in the Adult Life Course: Advocacy for Early Prevention," *Journal of Epidemiology and Community Health* 63 (June 2009): 563–68, http://www.ncbi.nlm.nih.gov/pmc/articles/PMC2696641.
7. P. T. Davies, et al., "Adrenocortical Underpinnings of Children's Psychological Reactivity to Interparental Conflict," *Child Development* 79, no. 6 (2008): 1693–706, http://www.ncbi.nlm.nih.gov/pubmed/19037943.
8. Marilynn Ellis, "Violent Home Is a War Zone for Kids," *USA Today*, 9 February 1999.
9. M. A. Straus, R. J. Gelles, and S. K. Steinmetz, *Behind Closed Doors: Violence in the American Family* (Garden City, NY: Doubleday, Anchor Press, 1980).
10. P. Jaffe and M. Sudermann, "Child Witness of Women Abuse: Research and Community Responses," in *Understanding Partner Violence: Prevalence, Causes, Consequences, and Solutions: Families in Focus Services*, Vol II, ed. S. Stith and M. Straus (Minneapolis, MN: National Council on Family Relations, 1995).

Chapter 9: Shelters

1. Texas Council on Family Violence, "Family Violence Statistics in Texas," June 2006, http://www.tcfv.org/pdf/dvam07/Year%202006%20Family%20Violence%20Statistics(HHSC).pdf.
2. Jessica Ashley, "Prostitution Study Finds Chicago Girls Trafficked Through Coercion, Violence," Research Bulletin, Illinois Criminal Justice Information Authority, September 2008, 2.
3. Ibid., 3.

Chapter 11: Lessons Learned from Survivors

1. Gavin De Becker, *The Gift of Fear* (New York: Bantam Doubleday Dell, 1998), 213.

Chapter 12: Building Alliances

1. Joan Zorza, "Woman Battering: A Major Cause of Homelessness," in *Clearinghouse Review* 25, no. 4 (1991): 421–27.
2. E. L. Bassuk, et al., "The Characteristics and Needs of Sheltered Homeless and Low-Income Housed Mothers," *Journal of the American Medical Association* 276, no. 8 (1996): 640–46.

Chapter 13: Lessons Learned Through Leading Domestic Violence Programs

1. Jim Collins, *Good to Great and the Social Sectors* (New York: HarperCollins, 2005), 5.

Chapter 14: Our Work Isn't Done

1. Colleen Newquist, "Bully Proof Your School," *Education World*, 2006, http://www.educationworld.com/a_admin/admin/admin018.shtml.
2. Barbara Ball and Barri Rosenbluth, "Expect Respect Program Overview" (SafePlace, Feb. 2008), 16.
3. National Women's Law Center, "I Am Not Worth Less" campaign, 2010, http://www.nwlc.org.
4. Evelyn F. Murphy, testimony before the US House of Representatives Subcommittee on Workforce Protections, Washington, DC, 11 July 2007.

⤳ *Resources* ⤳

To locate assistance in your community contact the National Domestic Violence Hotline at (800) 799-7233, TTY (800) 787-3224, or www.ndvh.org.

Helpful Organizations and Agencies

American Bar Association Commission on Domestic Violence
740 15th St. NW, Washington DC 20005
(202) 662-1000   www.abanet.org/domviol

Amnesty International USA, Women's Human Rights Program
322 8th Ave., New York NY 10001
(212) 633-4292   www.amnestyusa.org/women

Asian and Pacific Islander Institute on Domestic Violence
450 Sutter St., #600, San Francisco CA 94108
(415) 954-9988, ext. 315   www.apiahf.org/apidvinstitute

Bureau of Justice Statistics Clearinghouse
810 7th St. NW, Washington DC 20531
(800) 851-3420   www.ojp.usdoj.gov/bjs

Centers for Disease Control and Prevention
1600 Clifton Rd., Atlanta GA 30333
(800) 232-4636, TTY (888) 232-6348   www.cdc.gov

Child Welfare League of America
440 1st St. NW, 3rd Fl., Washington DC 20001
(202) 638-2952   www.cwla.org

Childhelp USA
15757 N. 78th St., Scottsdale AZ 85260
(800) 422-4453   www.childhelpusa.org

Children's Defense Fund
25 E St. NW, Washington DC 20001
(202) 628-8787   www.childrensdefense.org

Family Violence Prevention Fund
383 Rhode Island St., #304, San Francisco CA 94103
(415) 252-8900, TTY (800) 595-4889   www.endabuse.org

The Feminist Majority and the Feminist Majority Foundation
1600 Wilson Blvd., #801, Arlington VA 22209
(703) 522-2214
433 S. Beverly Dr., Beverly Hills CA 90212
(310) 556-2500   www.feminist.org

Human Rights Watch
350 5th Ave., 34th Fl., New York NY 10118
www.hrw.org

Institute on Domestic Violence and Sexual Assault
University of Texas School of Social Work,
1925 San Jacinto Blvd., Austin TX 78712
(512) 471-5457   www.utexas.edu/ssw/cswr/institutes/idvsa/

Institute on Domestic Violence in the African American Community
University of Minnesota School of Social Work, College of Human Ecology,
290 Peters Hall, 1404 Gortner Ave., St. Paul MN 55108
(877) 643-8222   www.dvinstitute.org

Jewish Women International
2000 "M" St. NW, #720, Washington, DC 20036
(800) 343-2823   www.jewishwomen.org

LAMBDA GLBT Community Services
216 S. Ochoa St., El Paso TX 79901
(206) 350-4283   www.lambda.org

The Miles Foundation (violence and the military)
PO Box 423, Newton CT 06470
(203) 270-7861   members.aol.com/milesfdn/myhomepage

National Center for Elder Abuse
1201 15th St. NW, #350, Washington DC 20005
(202) 898-2586   www.elderabusecenter.org

National Center for Victims of Crime
2000 M St. NW, Ste. 480, Washington DC 20036
(202) 467-8700   www.ncvc.org

National Clearinghouse on Child Abuse and Neglect Information
330 C St. SW, Washington DC 20447
(800) 394-3366   www.childwelfare.org

National Coalition for the Homeless
1012 14th St. NW, #600, Washington DC 20005
(202) 737-6444   www.nationalhomeless.org

National Domestic Violence Hotline
PO Box 161810, Austin TX 78716
(800) 799-7233, TTY (800) 787-3224   www.ndvh.org

National Health Resource Center on Domestic Violence
383 Rhode Island St., #304, San Francisco CA 94103
(888) 792-2873   www.endabuse.org

National Network to End Domestic Violence
660 Pennsylvania Ave. SE, #303, Washington DC 20003
(202) 543-5566   www.nnedv.org

National Organization for Victim Assistance
1730 Park Rd. NW, Washington DC 20010
(800) 879-6682   www.try-nova.org

National Resource Center on Domestic Violence—
Pennsylvania Coalition Against Domestic Violence
6400 Flank Dr., #1300, Harrisburg PA 17112
(800) 537-2238, TTY (800) 553-2508   www.nrcdv.org

National Runaway Switchboard
3080 N. Lincoln Ave., Chicago IL 60657
(773) 880-9860/(800) 621-4000   www.nrscrisisline.org

National Sexual Violence Resource Center
123 N. Enola Dr., Enola PA 17025
(877) 739-3895, TTY (717) 909-0715   www.nsvrc.org

National Teen Dating Abuse Helpline
(866) 331-9474, TTY (866) 331-8453   www.loveisrespect.org

National Women's Political Caucus
1634 Eye St. NW, #310, Washington DC 20006
(202) 785-1100   www.nwpc.org

Rape, Abuse & Incest National Network (RAINN)
2000 L St. NW, Suite 406, Washington DC 20036
(800) 656-4673, ext. 3   www.rainn.org

Resource Center on Domestic Violence: Child Protection & Custody—
National Council on Juvenile & Family Court Judges
PO Box 8970, Reno NV 89507
(800) 527-3223   www.nationalcouncilfvd.org

Sacred Circle—National Resource Center to End Violence
Against Native Women
722 Saint Joseph St., Rapid City SD 57701
(877) 733-7623

SafePlace
PO Box 19454, Austin TX 78760
(512) 267-7233, TTY (512) 927-9616   www.safeplace.org

Substance Abuse and Mental Health Services Administration (SAMHSA)
1 Choke Cherry Rd., Rockville MD 20857
(877) 726-4727, TTY (800) 487-4889   www.samhsa.gov

Violence Against Women Office, US Department of Justice
10th and Constitution Ave. NW, #5302, Washington DC 20530
(202) 616-8994   www.ojp.usdoj.gov/vawo

Helpful Training and Reading Materials

Akers, Dianne King, Wendie H. Abramson, and Michelle "Shell" Schwartz. *Balancing the Power: Creating a Crisis Center Accessible to People with Disabilities.* Austin, TX: SafePlace, 2005. http://www.safeplace.org.

Akers, Dianne King, Wendie H. Abramson, and Michelle "Shell" Schwartz. *Beyond Labels: Working with Abuse Survivors with Mental Illness Symptoms or Substance Abuse Issues.* Austin, TX: SafePlace, 2007. http://www.safeplace.org.

Akers, Dianne King, Iracema Mastroleo, Wendie Abramson, Michelle "Shell" Schwartz, Diane McDaniel Rhodes, and Heather Kamper. *Unlocking Accessibility: Effectively Serving People with Disabilities.* Austin, TX: SafePlace, 2010. http://www.safeplace.org.

Ball, Barbara, and Barri Rosenbluth. *Expect Respect Program Overview: A School-Based Program for Preventing Teen Dating Violence and Promoting Safe and Healthy Relationships.* Austin, TX: SafePlace, 2008. http://www.safeplace.org.

Ball, Barbara, Barri Rosenbluth, and Agnes Aoki. *Expect Respect Program Manual Part I: Support Group Curriculum and Facilitator Guide.* Austin, TX: SafePlace, 2008. http://www.safeplace.org.

Ball, Barbara, Randy Randolph, and Barri Rosenbluth. *Expect Respect Program Manual Part II: SafeTeens Youth Leadership Curriculum and Facilitator Guide.* Austin, TX: SafePlace, 2008. http://www.safeplace.org.

Brown, Sandra L. *Counseling Victims of Violence: A Handbook for Helping Professionals,* 2nd ed. Alameda, CA: Hunter House Inc., Publishers, 2007.

Hines, Denise A., and Kathleen Malley-Morrison. *Family Violence in the United States: Defining, Understanding, and Combating Abuse.* Thousand Oaks, CA: Sage Publications, 2005.

Hughes, Celia M., and Wendie H. Abramson. *Stop the Violence, Break the Silence Training Guide: Building Bridges Between Domestic Violence and Sexual Assault Agencies, People with Disabilities, Families and Caregivers.* Austin, TX: SafePlace, 2000. http://www.safeplace.org.

Jayne, Pamela. *Ditch That Jerk: Dealing with Men Who Control and Hurt Women.* Alameda, CA: Hunter House Inc., Publishers, 2000.

Lissette, Andrea, and Richard Kraus. *Free Yourself from an Abusive Relationship: Seven Steps to Taking Back Your Life.* Alameda, CA: Hunter House Inc., Publishers, 2000.

Robbi, Nelia J., Cema S. Mastroleo, and Wendie H. Abramson. *Responding to Violent Crimes Against Persons with Disabilities: A Manual for Law Enforcement, Prosecutors, Judges and Court Personnel.* Austin, TX: SafePlace, 2005. http://www.safeplace.org.

Rosenbluth, Barri, and Barbara Ball. *Expect Respect Program Manual Part III: School-wide Prevention Strategies Facilitator Guide and Resource.* Austin, TX: SafePlace, 2008. http://www.safeplace.org.

Wilson, K. J. *When Violence Begins at Home: A Comprehensive Guide to Understanding and Ending Domestic Abuse,* 2nd ed. Alameda, CA: Hunter House Inc., Publishers, 2006.

⌒ *Index* ⌒

HV
6626
.W484
2011